# ESCAPE ROOT

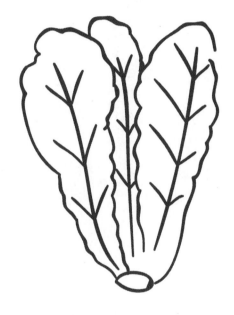

## THE SECRET PASSAGE TO

## LIFELONG WELLNESS

## SCOTT LAIRD, ND

Escape Root
The Secret Passage to Lifelong Wellness
By Scott Laird, ND

Paperback Edition, 1st printing
Copyright © 2017 Scott Laird

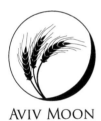

## AVIV MOON

Aviv Moon Publishing
PO Box 1559
Fort Mill, SC 29716
www.ARoodAwakening.tv

For questions or information regarding this publication, contact Aviv Moon Publishing at (888) 766-3610.

Graphic design: Brandon Randolph and Sterling Martin
Editing and proofing: R. Frank Bowers and Cat Everett

ISBN-10: 1979567093

Printed in the USA

# TABLE OF CONTENTS

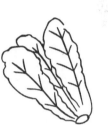
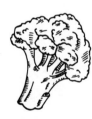

# FOREWORD

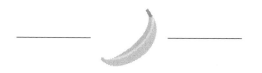

As a nutrition researcher, author, and adjunct associate professor of medicine at the George Washington University School of Medicine, I conduct studies on the role of nutrition in diabetes, obesity, and lipid management, among other health issues through The Physicians Committee for Responsible Medicine. The efforts of our 12,000 physician members are dramatically changing the way doctors treat chronic diseases such as diabetes, heart disease, obesity, and cancer, and empowering people to take control of their own health — Scott Laird shares this crucial mandate and mission.

Scott represents rare leadership in a new generation of wellness advocates. His passion to communicate the inspiring truth of self-healing is critical to continue the message of natural health information on which the future of young Americans rests.

The book you are about to read, "Escape Root: The Secret Passage to Lifelong Wellness" is especially important as it boils down complicated health and disease information into one of the relatively few sources of simplified, nutritional truth available to the general public. It will make you think and, I trust, inspire you to act upon what you read.

In short, this book represents your opportunity to take control of your health, to direct your health destiny, and to live in wellness for a lifetime.

Enjoy the read.

Neal Barnard, MD
President, The Physicians Committee for Responsible Medicine
pcrm.org

# INTRODUCTION

Is there truly an escape route (or "root" if you will)
that enables you to sidestep the disease statistics of
the modern world? Indeed there is, and it's simpler
than you might think. In fact, I've met hundreds of
people who have seen the symptoms of their life-
threatening diseases simply disappear after making
a simple diet change. In some cases, it took a year
or more; in others, less than a month. I've seen
diabetics reverse the symptoms of their condition in
as little as two weeks, and I interviewed a woman a
few years ago who reversed all symptoms of an egg-
sized breast cancer in just three months.

One interview I'll never forget was with a worship
pastor who had lost his ability to play the piano
because of multiple sclerosis. He had an MRI
at the time of his diagnosis that showed lesions
on his brain, confirming that his symptoms were
due to MS. He decided to forgo modern medical
treatments and adopt the diet discussed in this

book. One year later, having refused any medical treatments, he had another MRI. The lesions were gone and so were his symptoms. The doctor in charge of his care told him plainly, "You could quit your job right now and make a living going with me to every medical conference in the world to show them your before and after MRIs, because you have the proof that diet change alone can reverse symptoms of MS. Doctors have never seen that before."

I've seen symptom reversal from several diseases in my own family. Because of the diet we will discuss in the following pages, I no longer have acid reflux or heart palpitations. My wife has been able to bring hypothyroidism, or Hashimoto's Disease, under control. My parents, who both had colon cancer within three years of each other, have had perfectly clear colonoscopies since adopting the diet change — in their 70s! And my children, who both had asthma, no longer have any symptoms; all signs disappeared less than a month after giving up foods that were causing the problems. People look at me strangely when I tell them that my kids grew up on this diet. "Don't kids need more than that?" they ask. Apparently not. My daughter competed internationally as part of the Gymnastics Canada National Team and was subsequently awarded a four-year, full-ride athletic scholarship as a Division-1 NCAA gymnast. My son, also a gymnast, is a five-time all-around state champion. How can a diet change do all of this? Don't you need a special diet for this and a special diet for that? No! Why? Because the truth is that all disease is the same thing; it's just different manifestations. All disease is simply malfunctioning cells. And the best way to ensure that cells function properly, especially after they have malfunctioned, is with a plant-based diet.

The answers are not in the food, per se, but the right food does provide what the body needs to heal itself. Though modern times have blinded us to this fact, it's nothing new. In fact, the principles of a plant-based diet for everyday health and even reversal of disease are both in the very beginning of the Bible (in Genesis) and at the end (in Revelation). You may have never recognized it, but that's because we often short-change God's word by considering it only as a spiritual book, not a how-to manual for physical healing. But it really is. Let me explain what I mean.

Consider Genesis 1:29. This is the verse where, immediately after creating Adam, the first instruction God gives to mankind — yes, the FIRST and arguably most IMPORTANT instruction — is how to nourish the human body. He says:

> "See, I have given you every herb bearing seed (vegetables, legumes, grains, herbs and spices), which is on the face of all the earth, and every tree, which is the fruit of a tree yielding seed; to you it shall be for food."

Notice here that God does not say, "After you eat some plants, put that cow I just created into a corral, raise it, drink its milk, then kill its offspring, cut it up, roast it over fire, and eat it." He didn't even tell Adam to go fishing. The ONLY thing he instructed Adam to do for nourishment was to eat what grows from the ground.

Now, think about this for a moment. God loved Adam. He created Adam to be the ONLY being that was created in His likeness. Adam is His baby, His crown jewel, His masterpiece, the crescendo in the creation symphony. Obviously, he wants Adam to be healthy. And he's not going to forget to tell

Adam to eat something or deliberately wait and then add some more to the menu later. No. God, in his very first conversation with mankind, immediately and deliberately tells Adam what to eat in order to live and be healthy in one simple statement: raw, whole, plant-based foods.

It should come as no surprise that these plants are not just food, but medicine, too. Some of the greatest wisdom in natural medicine hasn't changed in thousands of years. The ancient physician Hippocrates, considered to be the father of medicine, said, "Let food be your medicine, and medicine your food." Native peoples from all over the world knew that nearby plants were the medicine for almost any ailment that they would experience living in that particular area.

We also see a hint of the same Genesis 1:29 instruction in the book of Revelation. Sometimes, we as followers of Messiah tend to over-spiritualize what's written in the Bible, but Revelation 22:2 says "The leaves of the trees are for the healing of the nations" – sure, it's a prophetic verse but it also has physical meaning.

Ashwagandha, for example, is a tropical herb used in Indian Ayurvedic medicine. It has a long history of health promoting and therapeutic effects and was the subject of an anticancer study in 2013. In the study, anticancer activity in the water extract of ashwagandha leaves was detected in both in vitro (test tube) and in vivo (living organism) tests. Researchers found that ashwagandha was "cytotoxic (toxic to living cells) to cancer cells selectively and causes tumor suppression" while "normal cells remained unaffected."[1] Similarly, the castor oil bean plant (Ricinus communis L.) — though the bean itself is one of the most poisonous plant substances in the world — yields an oil that has been used as a labor-inducer and laxative for centuries. Modern medical research has now also found that the oil in the leaves has medicinal potential, showing "strong antimicrobial activity" and "anticarcinogenic properties".[2]

In 2017, a study published in *Pharmaceutical Biology* (a monthly, peer-reviewed medical journal) evaluated the antioxidant potential of "bui" leaves found in arid regions of India. The study found that the leaves offer inflammatory relief from disorders associated with oxidative stress (i.e. rheumatic pain and healing of wounds) and "substantiates folk use of leaves in inflammatory disorders."[3] That statement is a major triumph for traditional, plant-based healing and, more importantly, gives a scientific nod to the biblical truth of Revelation 22:2. Modern science is now proving to us what ancient civilizations have always known: There are hundreds of trees and other plants whose leaves, roots, and other parts truly offer healing for anyone who will go back to the basics of the Almighty's Word to find healing for their body — including DNA repair. In fact, there have been at least 12 studies documented which clearly show that dietary factors influence the effectiveness of DNA repair.[4] Furthermore, research within the last few years has found that DNA repair "plays a crucial role in preventing cancer."[5]

The truth is, eating the right foods and proper nutritional supplementation has the potential to supercharge your body's own ability to repair your DNA, and at least 50 genetic-related diseases have responded favorably when the body is fed with essential nutrients.[6]

Yes, DNA repair is real. And to achieve it, all we need to do is get back to the basics.

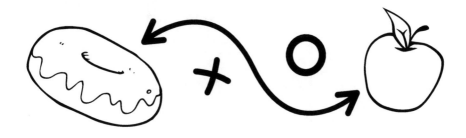

# PART 1

## SECRETS & STRATEGY

# THE TRUTH

> **Right foods heal. Wrong foods cause problems.**

The truth that no one is telling these days is that eating the right foods can not only prevent the symptoms of disease, but reverse them — and the power to do so comes from within the human body. A plant-based diet provides the body with the right combination to "turn on" this power, not only in times of healing, but every day. A plant-based diet can go a long way to keeping a person forever safe from the killer diseases that plague the Western world: heart disease, cancer, diabetes, arthritis, fibromyalgia, etc.

Most of today's feared diseases are simply imbalances caused over time, usually due to poor food choices. Food is our fuel; it's what makes us "go". Just like choosing the right fuel for your car, choosing what we eat determines whether our body operates the way it is supposed to. Choosing the right food is the single, most important health choice we make every day. Right foods heal. Wrong foods cause problems. Unfortunately, it's not always simple to identify what constitutes "good" food. There's money to be made in the food business and greed tends to cloud the truth. Clever number skewing, missing details and small survey samples can all be used to whitewash nutritional research findings so that they benefit a certain industry or company. Here's an example of how the deception works.

Let's say you have a cancer prevention drug trial including 100 participants and every one of the participants is administered the drug during the trial. The researchers make an assumption at the outset of the trial that two participants are likely to get cancer. By the conclusion of the trial, only one person actually gets cancer. If we look at this result from a logical point of view, this drug was only 1% effective because it only "prevented" cancer in one out of 100 people. This calculation is called an "absolute benefit". However, the drug company that sponsored the trial spent a lot of money and time on this trial. Furthermore, no one is going buy a drug that is only 1% effective. So, using the same numbers, but from a different perspective, the drug company will report things this way: Since two people were "expected" to get cancer, and the drug prevented cancer in one of those two people (i.e. 1/2), the drug is determined to be 50% effective. This is called a "relative benefit" and, completely legally, the drug can be marketed using this number. This example is derived from a revealing DVD by Mike Anderson, which I highly encourage you to view. It is called *Healing Cancer from Inside Out*.

Thankfully, smart consumers like you are not taking these findings at face value anymore. Universal internet access, social media sites, blogs, and other online forums have given us unprecedented access to research records and to the work of health advocates who are routinely blowing the whistle on bogus claims.

A typical example of this is a 2009 incident in which a children's breakfast cereal company plastered its cartoon-clad cereal boxes with the claim that the cereal now contained "A good source of calcium and vitamin D" and "Nutrition to help your kids grow up strong!" At face value, the claim was essentially true. Calcium and vitamin D will indeed help children grow up strong if, that is, these nutrients are derived from plant-based, whole food sources, which contain all of the naturally-occurring co-factors present in their natural state. Of course, in the case of refined, boxed breakfast cereal, this is not the case. Thus, the "healthy" claim was found to be disingenuous.

The whole truth in the case of breakfast cereal is that the amount of sugar and refined corn in the cereal completely nullify the amount of calcium and vitamin D added to it, not to mention that the calcium and vitamin D had to be artificially inserted into the cereal to make the claim. These nutrients are "isolated" nutrients, meaning they have been extracted from their natural state and separated from countless, complementary, naturally-occurring nutrients that help it carry out its expected benefits in the human body. These boxes of cereal are still on the shelves, but several blog posts and news reports have since exposed this half-truth to a wide audience.

Furthermore, refined sugar — regardless of how many "vitamins and minerals" accompany it in a breakfast cereal:

- *Suppresses the immune system*

- *Upsets the mineral relationships in the body*

- *Causes blood proteins to function less effectively*

- *Produces a significant rise in triglycerides which can contribute to juvenile delinquency and obesity in children*

- *Contributes to premature aging*

- *Aggravates arthritis, and is associated with the development of Parkinson's disease.*[7]

Don't forget that the milk served with the cereal has been sterilized of any perceived beneficial nutrients then "fortified" with artificial nutrients. Milk also contains animal-source protein, which has a list of issues all its own. Still want that crunchy, chocolaty bowl of disease?

Speaking of disease, we spend all kinds of time and money on disease research and therapeutic solutions, but cutting disease out or poisoning it or, more accurately, its symptoms, into submission is not the answer. We need to focus on examining the fuel that made the body break down in the first place and using better fuel to reverse the damage. As we have already established, that "breakdown" called disease, no matter what form it takes, is simply malfunctioning cells. And the reason cells malfunction is twofold: toxicity and deficiency. In other words, we get sick because we have too many toxins in our body and/or we are deficient in nutrients. (More on this later.)

# THE SECRET

The secret to attacking cellular malfunction is to address both toxicity and deficiency simultaneously. Many people choose to address toxicity (i.e. detox) with a

> A cleanse is very helpful, but motives must be examined before you begin.

"cleanse", such as consuming nothing but lemon juice, cayenne pepper, and maple syrup for a week or taking some capsule concoction out of a box from the health food store. Unless you are coupling that detox with a highly concentrated, pure, and easily assimilated form of nutrition, you may be doing more harm than good.

Don't get me wrong, a cleanse is very helpful, but motives (and methods) must be examined before you begin. Are you planning on changing the "fuel" you consume after you are done with the cleanse, or are you going to go right back to the same old dietary habits you had before the cleanse? If you're going to go back to your same old diet, what's the point? Are you clearing out as much of the junk as possible to give yourself an extended license to avoid changing your diet and lifestyle for just a little longer? (Be honest with yourself, now.) When people ask me if I think that they should do a colon cleanse or some other type of cleanse, I always tell them the same thing: I would not do it if I was not willing to improve my diet and lifestyle after the cleanse is complete. It defeats the purpose.

There's no sense going to the trouble of a cleanse and trudging through all the less-than-pleasant symptoms of a detoxification if it's not for the purpose of changing your life. Depending on how extreme your chosen cleanse method is and how ill-advised your diet has been for who-knows-how-long, you could have some pretty nasty detox symptoms (acne, dandruff, bad breath, foul waste, headaches, nausea, etc.) as your body is finally afforded the strength and opportunity to get rid of everything that has been impeding its ability to be as healthy as possible. A detox is a triumph! But without an improvement in your diet and lifestyle at the end of the process, all you're going to do is strip away the bad, which is a good thing, but then go right back to pouring in more junk. You're no further ahead than when you started. Not to mention, you're going to have to go through those same detox symptoms all over again the next time you decide to "cleanse".

> Half-way NEVER cuts it  in terms of faith, or good health.

Some health professionals say that a cleanse without an intentional improvement in diet and lifestyle puts one even further behind. This is because, once you strip away the junk, your body is in pristine condition, meaning that it can now absorb nutrients (and junk) better than ever. If, after your cleanse, you go right back to pouring bad food into a freshly cleaned body, it's going to be absorbed into your bloodstream even more efficiently than before, dragging you down even further (and faster).

It's a lot like the principles the Messiah taught about following Him: Don't bother if you're not willing to change your ways. Have you ever noticed His actions on this matter? He NEVER apologized for demanding repentance (i.e. changing one's ways). Think about any and every story in the Bible where He was teaching and preaching — not ONCE did He chase after someone who wasn't willing to live by His example. If someone wasn't willing to do what was necessary (like the rich young ruler - Luke 18:18-25), He essentially said, "OK, suit yourself.

> If you're a new creation, you're a new creation, not a new creation with a new supply of old habits that you have to purge all over again.

Good-bye!" Why? Because half-way NEVER cuts it in terms of faith, or good health. If you're a new creation, you're a new creation, not a new creation with a new supply of old habits that you have to purge all over again. That's not the idea of accepting Him and walking in His ways. And it's not the idea of a physical cleanse, either.

So, when you cleanse, use the opportunity to change your ways, and make sure to address toxicity and deficiency together. Use a cleansing method that incorporates concentrated, efficient nutrition that will supercharge your immune system. Once the body is armed with the nutrition it needs to not only maintain good health, but has an extra boost of power to tackle and expel stubborn toxins that have been hanging around for far too long (usually lurking in fat cells, your arteries, and in your digestive system), your body begins to heal itself. If you haven't seen self-healing like this before, it's because your body was simply not ready. It was not armed with what it needed to deploy the troops into battle.

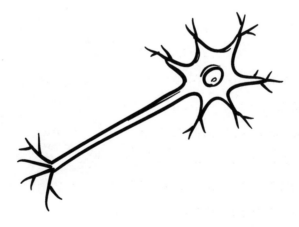

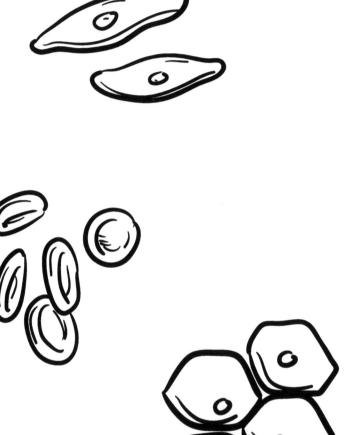

# LIFE BEGETS LIFE

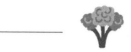

Life begets life — it's the definition of biogenesis (the production of a new, living organism), the most basic of biological principles on this earth, as demonstrated by the 1800s chemist Louis Pasteur. Pasteur's name is now a household term denoting high heat food preservation: "pasteurization." (Now, pasteurized food has its issues, as high heat destroys fragile, heat-sensitive nutrients, but we'll discuss that later.) In terms of biogenesis, Pasteur proved that living organisms are necessary to create similar organisms, rather than them spawning from nonliving matter, as was previously hypothesized.[8] In other words, living things provide life to other living things.

Dead things cannot provide life to living things. For example, it takes a living mother to give birth to a living baby. Ironically, most of us don't think about this "life begets life" principle when it comes to what we eat, yet "living" food — raw, whole, plant-based food — is the ideal way to provide "life" to our bodies. The life force in each raw, living plant creates a unique signature of enzymes, phytonutrients, minerals, and other nutrients. This signature creates an energy pattern that transfers the plant's living energy to the human body when consumed. However, cooking above temperatures of 122°F breaks down the plant's energy pattern, making it less effective and less beneficial.

Now, that doesn't mean that cooked food is useless to the human body. True, cooked food is devoid of living enzymes, but consuming a moderate amount of cooked, plant-based food is not a bad thing. In fact, it can be quite beneficial. Certain beneficial phytochemicals, such as lycopene and carotenoids, are activated by the cooking process; in addition, some proteins and starches are more readily available in cooked foods. Cooking does, however, destroy a significant percentage of a raw food's nutrients, such as vitamin C, along with ALL enzymes (no enzyme can survive when heated above

122°F).

On the other hand, eating ONLY raw, plant-based foods tends to limit one's food choices. Dr. Joel Fuhrman, a well-known, staunch advocate of a primarily raw, plant-based diet comments, "To exclude all steamed vegetables and vegetable soups from your diet narrows the nutrient diversity of your diet and has a tendency to reduce the percentage of calories from vegetables, in favor of nuts and fruits, which are lower in nutrients per calorie. Unfortunately, sloppy science prevails in the 'raw food' movement."

However, the fact remains that raw foods are, in more ways than not, superior as they have their own enzymes (life force); each raw, uncooked fruit, vegetable, nut, or seed contains enzymes that will digest the food in which they are contained. Cooked foods (and processed foods) are devoid of enzymes and thus rely on your body's own pancreatic enzymes for digestion — the more your body has to generate its own enzymes, the more stressed it becomes.

The idea becomes obvious: Get more living food into your body. In fact, if you get enough living (i.e. raw) food into your body to address deficiencies while getting rid of toxins at the same time, you can actually turn the tide of disease symptoms. Symptoms of cancer, for example, can and do disappear this way. Symptoms of clogged arteries disappear this way. Symptoms of painful deposits in joints and bones dissolve this way. Even symptoms of emotional and neurological disorders can be lessened or even halted altogether. All you have to do is provide the body what it needs to do the job.

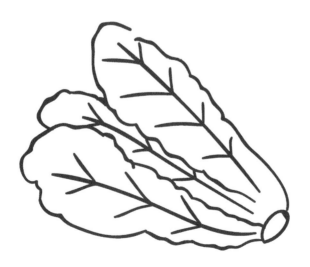

# THE ULTIMATE WELLNESS WEAPON

Nutrition — concentrated nutrition — is the key to health; this is why so many nutritional supplements have been introduced in recent years. But raw, whole, plant-based foods are still the best because they contain a complete profile of natural compounds that work in synergy as nature intended. Isolated nutrients developed into a supplement can help give the body a boost, but can never have the same, superior synergy that matches the human body's complex need for nutrients found in their natural state, accompanied by all of the cofactors that make each nutrient function to their maximum God-given capacity.

Freshly extracted, raw vegetable juices are the ultimate expression of this synergy — they are the best of the best. They provide the most amount of living food nutrition with the least amount of digestive effort from your body because the juice has been separated from the fiber, enabling the body to get much more nutrition to the cellular level much quicker and with much less energy. This allows your body to rest while arming it with the nutrients it needs to address deficiency, thereby enabling it to detoxify and fight the symptoms of disease. In effect, you are addressing toxicity and deficiency simultaneously. This is why juicing is the ultimate wellness weapon.

Let's use the example of a carrot to explain how this works. In his book, *Live Food Juices*, H.E. Kirschner, M.D., explains:

> "… the power to break down the cellular structure of raw vegetables, and assimilate the precious elements they contain, even in the healthiest individual is only fractional – not more than 35%, and in the less healthy, down to 1%. In the form of juice, these same individuals assimilate up to 92% of these elements… It is a well-known fact that all foods must become liquid before they can be assimilated."

In other words, even if your digestive system is healthy, you can only assimilate about 35%

(maximum) of the nutrition in a whole carrot. Your body has to break down the fiber of the carrot to get at the nutrients inside the carrot's cells. But if you use a juicer to separate the carrot's fiber from its juice and drink the juice, which contains the vast majority of the carrot's nutrients, all the work of breaking down the food into liquid has already been done. Instead of assimilating 35% of nutrition from a whole carrot, your body can now assimilate up to 92% of the nutrients from that same carrot by drinking the juice alone.

"Nature's medicines are locked in the cells of growing plants and released in their juices…These juices, subtle in their action yet more potent than any medicine, and without the toxic effect of drugs, can eliminate or prevent many of the chronic and degenerative diseases with which human beings are afflicted."

*- Drink Your Troubles Away*, by John Lust

In this example, you can get the nutrition of a pound of carrots in just eight ounces of juice; that's the kind of concentrated nutrition your body needs to reverse the symptoms of disease! Incidentally, when purchasing carrots for juicing, look for organic

California juicing carrots. They are usually much sweeter than those grown in other parts of the country because of the high trace mineral content of the soil.

It is important to remember that, to obtain the optimum nutrients, fresh juice should be consumed as quickly as possible after extracting it. Juice can also be stored in the refrigerator for a day or two; fill a resealable jar to the brim and seal tightly to avoid exposing the juice to air and light.

Of course, juicing organic produce is always the best choice, but if doing so is beyond your budget, make sure to remove as much of the pesticides and herbicides from your produce as possible.

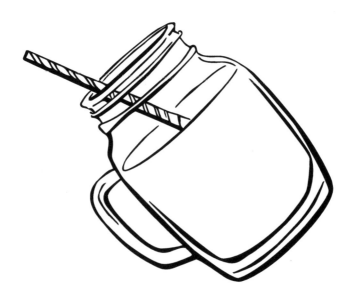

Dr. Michael Donaldson of The Hallelujah Diet shared this two-step produce washing process with me. It involves two spray bottles: one filled with distilled vinegar and another filled with food grade hydrogen peroxide:

1. **Spray the produce with the distilled vinegar** first to set up an acid environment to allow the peroxide to work more efficiently.

2. Then spray with **hydrogen peroxide**.

3. Let stand **4 to 5 minutes**.

4. **Rinse** thoroughly.

Juicing is vital no matter your age or physical condition because, whether you're sick or well, everyone's body replaces cells at

> Food is your fuel, so always choose "premium" fuel.

the rate of 300 million every minute. Obviously, every one of those 300 million cells that dies must be replaced with a new cell. What many people fail to realize, however, is that the quality of the replacement cells depends on the quality of food you are providing to your body — remember, food is your fuel, so always choose "premium" fuel.

If the quality of a new cell is better than the old one, the body can heal — this is how symptoms of disease are reversed — and juicing is the best source of high quality nutrition the body can get. Juicing enables the body to accomplish this miracle because it floods the body with concentrated, alkaline-forming nutrition. Why is this important? Because disease cannot thrive in an alkaline environment.

My parents, whom I mentioned in the introduction of this book, are a prime example of the amazing power juicing affords the human body. In 2001, I received a call from my parents with some bad news: Dad, age 66, was diagnosed with colon cancer. The good news was that the cancer had not spread beyond the colon wall and the doctors were confident that they could "get it all" by cutting out a small portion of his colon. He would not need radiation or chemotherapy, nor would he need a colostomy bag. Surgery went ahead and, to make a long story short, he recovered and everything was fine. He went for annual check-ups including a colonoscopy each year, during which the physician would find and remove suspect polyps for testing. (Polyps are precancerous growths stemming from the mucous membrane in the colon.) Each year, Mom and Dad would wait nervously and pray about the test results. Thankfully, each year the results were negative. However, he still worried about the cancer coming back.

Mom is three years younger than Dad. Like clockwork, three years after Dad's cancer ordeal, I received another call. Mom had the very same cancer Dad endured at age 66 three years prior, same diagnosis, same treatment, same outcome, and the same annual colonoscopies. Mom's cancer was in 2004, four years before I knew anything about natural health and healing. But even then I knew there was something odd going on. How could two people, from two totally different ends of the genetic spectrum, who grew up hundreds of miles away from each other, get the same cancer at the same age? Four years later, once I learned the truth that diet and lifestyle control genetic expression, it finally dawned on me — it had nothing to do with their genes. Mom and Dad endured the same cancer at the same age because they had been eating the same diet together for more than three decades.

Once I learned about the power of juicing and a plant-based diet, I began to educate my parents during our weekly phone calls. They have always been very curious and willing to support my career no matter what I was doing or where I was doing it. Eventually, I convinced them to buy a juicer and just "see what happens" if they adopted a primarily raw, plant-based diet and drink 16 ounces of carrot juice each day. Giving up meat was a little difficult, but they wanted to give the "plant-based thing" a fair shot. So, they persevered. Before long, they noticed an uptick in energy, more consistent and healthful bathroom trips, and a new zest for life in their retirement years.

After about a year of enjoying their new carrot juice routine, the true test came — their annual colonoscopies. For the first time in their lives — even before the cancer diagnoses — their colonoscopies were polyp-free. Not a growth to be found. They were sold! Today, nearly a decade later, they still drink carrot juice every day, mixed with raw, enzymatically alive beet juice powder and barley grass juice powder. They eat a primarily plant-based diet (unless friends invite them over for an occasional prized roast) and ensure they have a quarter cup of ground flax seed each morning (for regularity and omega 3 fatty acids, which we will discuss later). No one ever believes them when they reveal their age — because they're renewing their cells. They're doing something different than their peers, which is exactly why they look and feel younger than their peers.

Granted, if a person is juicing a quart of vegetable juice or more every day, it can cost a fair amount of money, especially if one is trying to do everything organic. It's not as expensive as chemotherapy or having a stent put in the heart, but expensive nonetheless. But here's my little money-saving secret: Most chemicals used on conventional produce are hydrophobic. That means they stick to the pulp of the fruits and vegetables, not the juice. And since juicing separates the fiber from the juice, there is a lot less exposure to these chemicals that one might think. However, it's still a good idea to wash everything first.

So what do you juice? First of all, it should be obvious that you can't just go out to the grocery store and buy juice off the shelf. Even expensive, organic vegetable juices in the refrigerated section of your grocery store won't help the body heal the way living food can. Why? If juice is on the shelf, the law says it has to be preserved (i.e. pasteurized). Pasteurization uses high temperatures to kill a vast majority of the raw food living enzymes. This is counterproductive because enzymes help the body improve cells, reverse symptoms of disease, and promote anti-aging.

> Pasteurization uses high temperatures to kill a vast majority of the raw food living enzymes. This is counterproductive because enzymes help the body improve cells, reverse symptoms of disease, and promote anti-aging.

And don't let the term "flash pasteurized" fool you. The food has still been heated. Now, pasteurized products are not all bad. They may have a fair bit of nutrition left in them, but it's not what is found in nature. Even "high pressure processing" is not the answer. With juicing popularity skyrocketing in recent years, some juice manufacturers employ this method by which juice is subjected to high pressures to keep it from spoiling. It's one step better than pasteurization since it does not involve heat, but the pressure still nullifies any "good" bacteria. Enzyme content is questionable as well, since one of the effects of high pressure processing is denaturing proteins to prevent spoilage, and enzymes are proteins.

What about juicing fruit? Raw fruit does indeed have living enzymes, but it's best consumed as a whole food, its fiber intact. Here's why: Part of the function of fiber in a whole piece of fruit is to regulate the release

> Drinking fiber-free juice on an empty stomach is best for shuttling nutrients directly to your cells to promote healing.

of the fruit's sugar in the bloodstream. When fruit is run through a juicer, the fiber is separated from the juice, which concentrates all of the sugar from that whole piece of fruit into a small amount of juice. Without the fiber to regulate it, the sugar is released into the bloodstream too quickly, and that's not conducive to healing.

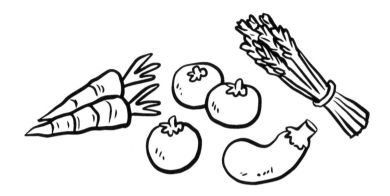

Vegetables, on the other hand, are the best thing to juice to get maximum nutrients into the body with the least amount of digestive effort; which, as you remember, promotes healing. Vegetables contain the 'building blocks' that develop powerful, healthy muscles, tissues, glands, and organs.

While all fruits and vegetables are important to maintain good health, some are exceptionally beneficial. Carrot juice, for example, makes a great base for all vegetable juices. Dark leafy greens such as spinach, parsley, kale, and leaf lettuce are extremely high in nutrients, and taste delicious when juiced with carrots. Vegetables, especially green leafy vegetables, have high vitamin and mineral content and not nearly the sugar of fruit. This is why raw, living vegetable juices are your most powerful form of healing. So, remember this rule of thumb: Eat your fruits, juice your vegetables.

Consider juice from living foods as your between-meals multivitamin. Indeed, raw vegetable juice is a much more effective and powerful multivitamin than anything that comes in tablet – 90% of those are a waste of money anyway. Now, "what about fiber?" you may be be asking. "Why would I remove all the fiber in juice? I thought fiber was good for the colon." Fiber is, indeed, good for the colon. And that's why, at meal times, you need lots of fiber in the form of raw, living foods on your plate. However, drinking fiber-free juice on an empty stomach is best for shuttling nutrients directly to your cells to promote healing; that's why it's so important to do so between meals. Without fiber to digest, the nutrients in raw, living juices can be delivered to your bloodstream almost immediately. Remember, food must be converted to liquid before your body can use it. Freshly extracted vegetable juice is already in liquid form, resulting in minimal stress to the immune system.

When someone adopts a primarily raw, plant-based diet as part of a strategy to reverse the symptoms of cancer, it is common to consume up to 12 cups of freshly extracted vegetable juice every day — one cup every waking hour aside from meal digestion times. Why? When the body is flooded with the superior, hyper-assimilated nutrients it needs to generate superior cells, the immune system is afforded the strength to gain the upper hand against the symptoms of disease.

# THE ULTIMATE WEIGHT-LOSS WEAPON

To lose weight and keep it off, just like reversing the symptoms of disease, the body needs a flood of alkaline-forming foods (juicing is the best way) and fewer acidic foods. Best of all, if a person's diet includes a variety-packed, plant-based diet of living foods in their natural state (i.e., primarily raw vegetables, vegetable juices, fruits, nuts, and seeds), calorie counting becomes irrelevant. The body will feel full long before consuming too many calories because plant-based foods are naturally high in nutrients, low in calories, and have fiber to make the body feel full. In other words, eating plant-based foods is self-limiting. It's exactly what the body needs, no more and no less, which is why it makes weight loss (and weight maintenance) effortless! Unfortunately, the "Standard American Diet" is riddled with the opposite: Low nutrient foods that are high in calories.

Consider this: If a person ate two apples (190 calories), three cups of boiled kale (84 calories), one cup of raw alfalfa sprouts (46 calories), and two ounces of walnuts (183 calories), they would be stuffed full of food that is loaded with fiber and a wealth of easily digested, immune-boosting nutrients and only 503 calories[9] — that's less than just one, medium-sized McCafe Mocha Frappe from McDonald's (560 calories). [10]

It's ironic, isn't it? The unhealthiest foods with the most calories have the least amount of nutrition per calorie, leaving the body starved for nutrients. This conundrum tells the brain to eat even more to fill the nutrient void — the perfect recipe for obesity. And once a person has started on a path to obesity, it can be hard to break the habit. Yes, obesity is indeed a result of habit; genes have relatively very little to do with whether a person is obese. That may be difficult to accept, but really, it's good news; it means that a person is not doomed to obesity just because their parents were. Even if a person has a genetic tendency to be overweight, individual diet

..................................

Even if a person has a genetic tendency to be overweight, individual diet and lifestyle choices are still the dominant factor in determining whether those genes get turned on or off (genetic expression)..

..................................

and lifestyle choices are still the dominant factor in determining whether those genes get turned on or off (genetic expression). Bottom line: Diet and lifestyle control genetic expression. And the best choices for diet have been known since the Garden of Eden. Like a textbook from heaven, the Bible is God's instruction manual to His children. It shows us both physical and spiritual truth for living our lives, including how to nourish our physical bodies for optimal health — without which we cannot effectively fulfill our spiritual duties! In fact, in God's very first instructions to human beings after He created us in the Garden of Eden, He told us what to eat:

"Then God said, "I give you every seed-bearing plant on the face of the whole earth and every tree that has fruit with seed in it. They will be yours for food."
- Genesis 1:29
If God's very first instructions to man were about food, it should be obvious to us that the human body

operates most efficiently on food he told us to eat, namely a primarily raw, plant-based diet as per the principles found in the Garden of Eden (Genesis 1:29). After all, it's God's original, perfect plan for our nourishment; and it still works today. In fact, the vast majority of people find that when they adopt a well-balanced, plant-based diet — high in fresh vegetables, low in processed foods (if any), plus a moderate intake of fresh, whole fruits, nuts, and seeds — they are able to achieve and maintain their ideal weight.

> Obesity, like disease, is simply cellular malfunction. Cells malfunction because of an imbalance of death and life in the body: Too much death, not enough life.

And the best part? When they lose the weight, all of their other physical problems (associated with excess toxins the body had been holding on to in the form of fat) simply melt away and their health is restored.

So, obesity, like disease, is simply cellular malfunction. Cells malfunction because of an imbalance of death and life in the body: Too much death, not enough life. That death is caused by poor food and lifestyle choices which cause oxidative stress, which leads to increased free radical activity in the body, which promotes disease. A free radical is a molecule that lacks an electron, making it unstable and damaging to the body as it hunts for an electron to "rob" from another molecule in order to regain its stability. Every time a molecule is robbed of an electron, it causes cellular damage. Alternatively, antioxidants in raw fruits and vegetables help to stop this process. Every antioxidant contains an **extra** electron in its molecular structure with the express purpose of "donating" that extra electron to a free radical molecule in order to stabilize it, thereby halting its damaging behavior.

A practical way to prove this concept to yourself is with exercise. Exercise creates excess oxidation, but if you restrict yourself to a primarily raw, plant-based diet between workouts, you'll notice that you're ready for your next workout much sooner than if you eat a regular diet. This is because you are flooding your body with antioxidants that help to stop damage induced by the oxidation caused by exercise. This is exactly why many world-class athletes are now getting on the plant-based bandwagon. Since plant-based foods help their body recover faster between workouts, they can improve their performance faster than their competitors by scheduling more workouts closer together.

As much as we try, we can't stop ALL oxidation; it happens with every metabolic process in the body. It happens with exercise. It even happens with breathing and thinking. The key is to counteract it as much as possible by ensuring that most of your diet consists of raw, living foods that have antioxidants your body needs to reverse the damage and the living enzymes that produce "life" for your living body.

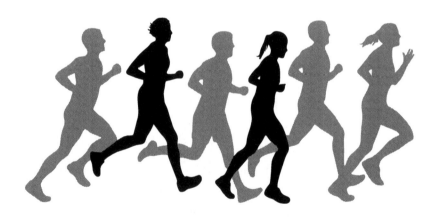

# DO WHAT NOBODY ELSE IS DOING

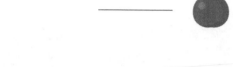

The bottom line is that a diet of plant-based, whole foods (primarily raw) has the God-given power to both rebuild your body's self-healing ability (so that your body can reverse symptoms of disease) and to maintain that state so disease cannot develop again. I know, I know. You don't want to be one of those weird, sandal-wearing, beard-growing, dreadlock-sporting, earth-worshipping, PETA-card-carrying "raw-foodists". And heaven forbid that you should even announce to your friends that you are simply "vegan". It's not what the rest of the world is doing. And that's exactly why you SHOULD be doing it (minus the sandals, beard, dreadlocks, ill-advised religious practices, and PETA membership, unless you like sandals, beards, and dreads).

In all seriousness, when your diet and lifestyle are healthier than the world around you, suddenly the world's statistics don't apply to you. Think about it: A statistic that says that "1 in 'x' Americans will get stuck in an elevator in their lifetime" doesn't apply to you if you never use an elevator. Likewise, a

> When your diet and lifestyle are healthier than the world around you, suddenly the world's statistics don't apply to you.

statistic that claims "1 in 'x' Americans will develop 'this or that' disease" is derived from a sample of typical Americans from all walks of life who may or may not be watching their diet and lifestyle. If you are one of the rare ones actually looking after your health and lifestyle in a way that the rest of that sample group is not, then you are not part of that statistic, and the results do not apply to you. This is powerful, so let me repeat that. If you're doing something different, something better than everyone else, you've taken yourself out of the equation. Those scary 'diseases-of-affluence' statistics will NOT apply to you.

In essence, when you decide to take care of your health in a "weird," yet extremely protective and empowering way, you change the game. Because you literally ARE what you EAT. Your body will indeed be different than those around you. Your cells will be more vibrant and resistant to the symptoms of disease because you are fueling them with foods jam-packed with life-giving force, and that gives you a health advantage. The way your body responds to everyday lifestyle factors is significantly superior when you choose to eat a high percentage of raw, living, plant-based foods and juices because your body is properly equipped to deal with the situation instead of succumbing to disease.

Let's take the example of being outside in the sunshine (without burning). When you're out in the sun, you are exposing your skin, which is your body's largest organ. And just like any other organ, your skin's ability to resist oxidation and disease depends on what you eat, because everything you eat eventually makes its way to your organs, including your skin. That's why the symptoms of skin conditions like eczema and psoriasis can often be corrected with diet change; more often than not, these symptoms are simply a result of the body reacting to an improper diet. It is trying to push out the toxins in any way it can, including through the skin. Now, if everything you eat makes its way to your skin, and if you eat a diet like everyone else (full of foods that do not equip the body's cells to protect themselves), you will render your skin defenseless against the oxidizing rays of the sun because the cells are ill-prepared to deal with the threat. This, in turn, causes them to malfunction, leading to diseases like skin cancer. But when you eat a diet rich in raw, living foods loaded with antioxidants, every organ in your body, including your skin, is well equipped to reverse oxidative damage. So, instead of malfunctioning when the sun hits your skin, your skin knows exactly what to do. It absorbs the UVB rays from the sun and uses the beneficial oils in your skin (derived from eating proper foods) to convert cholesterol into pre-vitamin D3, which benefits your entire body.

Contrary to the advice we've heard all our lives, it turns out that the best times to absorb beneficial UVB rays seem to be between 10:00am and 2:00pm when the UV index is above 3. Granted, when the sun is directly overhead, you must also be extra diligent not to burn. Outside of these prime hours, when the sun's rays are at an angle that forces them to pass through more of the atmosphere, a greater percentage of rays will be absorbed into the atmosphere. This means that less sunlight is absorbed into your skin and, ultimately, less vitamin D is created.

To this point, in April 2017, The Vitamin D Society of Canada published a press release, noting:

"Canadian vitamin D levels have dropped by 10% over the past six years. The root cause of this decrease is lower sun exposure. People are just not getting outside around midday in the summer and making vitamin D, and when they are outside they are using sunscreen, which, if applied correctly, prevents 95%+ of vitamin D production."

Furthermore, the press release noted:

"12 million citizens (35% of the total Canadian population) have vitamin D blood levels below the recommendations from Health Canada (an agency similar in function to the U.S. Department of Health and Human Services). This fact puts these people at a higher risk for several diseases, including cardiovascular disease, cancer, osteoporosis, diabetes, multiple sclerosis, Alzheimer's disease and many more. In fact, a study completed in 2016 reported that if Canadians increased their vitamin D levels to the recommended level of 100 nmol/L, we would save $12.5B in healthcare costs and 23,000 premature deaths annually. A recent study reported that women who avoided the sun have twice the risk of all-cause death. The authors said that "avoidance of sun exposure is a risk factor for death of a similar magnitude as smoking."

What about skin cancer? The press release had something to say about that, too:

"Research has shown that people with higher sun exposure such as outdoor workers, who have 3-10 times the sun exposure as indoor workers, have a lower incidence of melanoma. The National Cancer Institute reports that melanoma risk is increased as a result of intermittent acute sun exposure leading to sunburn."

Again, do what no one else is doing and your results will be different. This goes for digestion, too. Far too many people have digestive troubles today; and that's not just a concern for bloating, gas, and discomfort. Your body is not going to get much benefit from anything you eat if you have digestive troubles, because proper digestion is an important key to healing. In most cases, raw food is easiest for digestion because raw foods have their own enzymes to help the food break down and metabolize. However, people with irritable bowel syndrome, colon cancer, or stomach issues often have trouble digesting all of the raw food we've talked about. In fact, many doctors will tell people in this situation that they can't have raw food at all. Yet these folks have found another way to benefit from raw food — they juice it.

Since most of the nutrition in raw food is found in the juice, many people have found that a cup of juice every hour, day after day, helps the digestive system to heal. Then, once healing begins, a person with digestive issues can usually begin to include raw foods that have been blended in a blender. Why put raw food in a blender? Blended food is much easier to digest because the blender has done much of the digestion work already. Blending breaks open the cells of the food in a much more efficient way than chewing, and as a result, it's easier on your digestive system. Breaking open those cells also means that more nutrition is released, ensuring that you don't miss out on any of the value the food has to offer.

. . . . . . . . . . . . . . . . . . . . . . . . . . . . . . . . . . . . . . . . .

DID YOU KNOW?
Blended food can deliver as much as seven times the amount of nutrition of food chewed in its whole form.

. . . . . . . . . . . . . . . . . . . . . . . . . . . . . . . . . . . . . . . . .

Quite often, the very reason a person has any illness at all is because they're not absorbing nutrients, even if a digestive-related illness has never been diagnosed. You can have the greatest diet in the world, but if your body cannot absorb what you are eating, your great diet is null and void. Remember, toxicity and deficiency go hand in hand as the perfect recipe for disease. If you have toxins in your body (as everyone does), but you don't have the nutrient absorption to fight back (i.e. deficiency), you're headed for trouble.

One way to assist your body's digestion efficiency is to eat raw, unprocessed food. When a natural food with an unchanged, natural flavor comes into contact with your taste buds, your body will recognize the food and automatically secrete a special combination of digestive fluids that are best adapted to digest the specific food your taste buds are detecting.[11] This ensures that appropriate and efficient digestion starts on the right track, summoning pre-digestive juices in the mouth before the food reaches the stomach where the digestive "heavy lifting" takes place.

Alternatively, cooking or other processing changes the flavor of natural food; as a result, taste buds do not recognize the food, which sends a misguided message to the body and leads to a dysfunction in digestive fluid secretion.

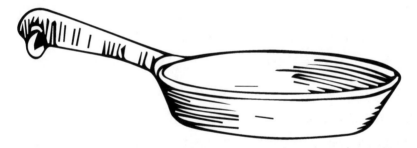

Nutrient absorption and gut health is not a new understanding. Thousands of years ago, Hippocrates (known as the father of medicine and from whose name we get "The Hippocratic Oath") stated, "All disease begins in the gut." Even in his day, he recognized the importance of gut health; indeed, gut health affects overall health. A visual example of this concept is an eye chart used in the natural health practice of iridology. Iridology examines the iris of the eye as a health map of the entire body. When illustrated on paper, the iris health map mimics the design of the eye, looking like the hub and spokes of a bicycle wheel — the hub being the pupil and the spokes being the iris, the colored part of the eye. Each section of the iris represents a particular part of the body, much like the nerve endings in the sole of the foot correspond to parts of the body.

Discolorations in a particular part of the iris indicate disharmony in the corresponding part of the body. For example, a dark spot in the lower left quadrant of the left eye indicates trauma or less-than-optimal function in the person's left kidney. While every other part of the body likewise occupies a small space in the spokes of the iridology map, there is one part of the body that affects the function of all others: The gut. On the iridology map, the gut is wrapped around the entire pupil, meaning that gut health affects all other "spokes" stemming from it.

For many reasons, the gut is indeed the command

center for human health. It is a fascinating warzone, a seesaw between good bacteria and pathogenic bacteria. The trick is to keep the seesaw balanced, lest pathogenic bacteria take more than their fair share of space in the gut and ruin the health of the host (i.e. you). The good bacteria/bad bacteria tug-of-war is a like a spaghetti western showdown at high noon: "There ain't room in this town (gut) for both of us!" There is only so much room for bacteria in the gut, so the good bacteria is either winning or losing at every moment of every day.

Many factors in today's world can lead to bacteria imbalance, which is why supplemental probiotics have become so popular. Probiotics help to address digestive bacteria imbalance; a proper balance of good bacteria and pathogenic bacteria is absolutely essential to be able to absorb nutrients and for the body to heal itself of disease.

One of the more eyebrow-raising gut bacteria discoveries in recent years is the role that animal-based foods (meat, eggs, dairy) play when it comes to cancer risk. The surprising thing about this discovery is that cancer risk does not come directly from the animal-based food itself (or even the fat of said foods). The problem arises in the process by which the human body digests it. When the human body's intestinal bacteria digest red meat, eggs, and dairy, the liver responds by producing a substance called trimethylamine-N-oxide (TMAO). High levels of this compound in a person's blood are now considered to be the "smoking gun" for colon cancer risk.

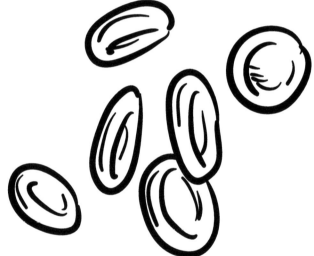

Specifically, a five-year study showed that women with the highest level of TMAO in their blood plasma had the highest risk for rectal cancer — up to 340% greater risk than women with the lowest TMAO levels![12] In other words, avoid these foods and you will avoid the alteration of your gut bacteria and thus avoid the risk of colorectal cancer associated with such alteration. Another study, which focused solely on egg consumption, widened the disease risk of elevated TMAO levels to include breast, ovarian, and prostate cancers. The study stated, "High egg intake (five eggs or more per week) may be associated with a modestly elevated risk of breast cancer, and a positive association between egg intake and ovarian and fatal prostate cancers cannot be ruled out."

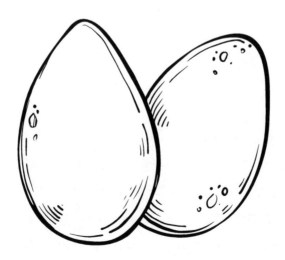

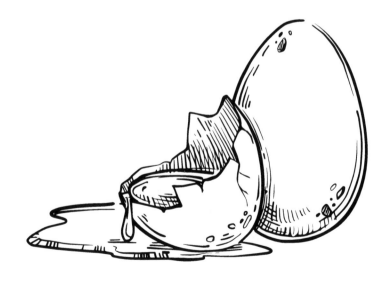

# HOW TO MAKE THE RIGHT CHOICES

Now, we've talked a lot about the importance of proper food, digestion, and absorption. It's time to get into the details of what comprises your food, what each component does, and to give you a greater understanding of WHY it is so important to make the right choices. We've also spent time favoring "a primarily raw, plant-based diet". So just how much raw food are we talking about here?

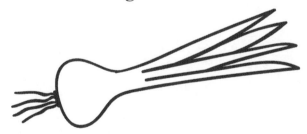

The ideal scenario, in my experience, is about 80% to 85% raw food and 15% to 20% cooked (all plant-based, of course). Why not 100% raw food? First of all, it's pretty challenging to do a 100% raw diet (even if you're a single person with lots of time to do your own thing). Secondly, there are some benefits to cooked food even though some of the nutrients are destroyed in cooking and/or processing. Cooked food helps some people feel fuller longer, and helps prevent rapid weight loss in people who don't have weight to lose.

But don't worry about making your cooked food portion exactly 15% or 20%; that's going to vary from person to person anyway. An easy way to make sure you're on track is to make every meal and every snack raw throughout the day, then add a cooked and/or processed food portion to only one meal after you've finished eating all the raw food first.

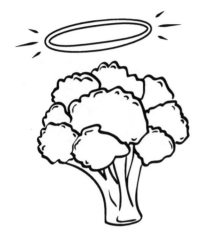
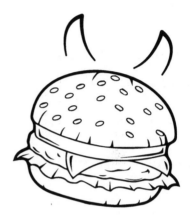

# >>> PART 2 <<<

## ALLIES & ENEMIES

# INTRODUCTION

Somehow, we've forgotten how to live the way the Almighty told us. We have lost sight of the simple instructions given to us at the beginning: Eat foods that grow from the ground, marry once for life, obey the Almighty's commands, etc. You know, simple stuff. Fortunately, just as there is a simple solution to coming back to righteous living after giving in to a wretched life, there is a simple solution to reversing the symptoms that make you feel tired and old. You can indeed restore your health to the very best it can be, for as long as possible.

In short, there really is a secret passage, if you will, to lifelong wellness. It starts with how you choose foods and educating yourself so that you can understand what you read on the back of food packages. We're going to cover a lot of the basics here. You may know much of this already, but I'm willing to bet you will also be have a few "ah-ha" moments, too. Let's start with some words that we "think" we know. Take the word "vitamin," for example.

# WHAT IS A VITAMIN?

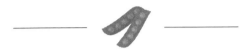

What is a vitamin? You've heard the term a million times, but what does it really mean? The official definition is, "a substance that is essential for normal cell function, growth, and development." Period. That's what a vitamin is. Seriously, *that's it*. And that's the point I'm trying to make here. Sometimes we shortchange ourselves because we don't educate ourselves about our own health. We've brainwashed ourselves into thinking that "you have to be an expert" to do anything about your own health, that such things are reserved for doctors and scientists.

Certainly, there are experts in the field, but each of us is responsible for our own health, and being smart about health is not as difficult as you might assume. Here is a crash course on vitamins to give you the basics: There are 13 essential vitamins. The word "essential" in this context means that the human body cannot manufacture them autonomously; essential vitamins can only be derived from food. Four of the 13 essential vitamins are fat soluble, which means that they are absorbed by fat globules in the human body; excesses are stored in the liver and fat tissues in case of a shortage. The fat soluble vitamins are A, D, E and K.

The other nine vitamins are water soluble. The human body absorbs and uses water soluble vitamins but it cannot store them; excess water soluble vitamins are simply excreted during bathroom breaks. For example, if you've ever taken a B vitamin complex, you may have noticed that your urine is bright yellow. This does not mean that your body is wasting the vitamin supplement. It means that your required vitamin B2 is topped up, and the excess is being pushed out. (B2 is known as the "yellow" vitamin; it is actually used for food coloring. B2 is also essential for creating red blood cells and for promoting cell growth, and is necessary for healthy muscle, nerve, and heart function.)

Incidentally, all B vitamins are water soluble, as is vitamin C. If a person has taken too much vitamin C, they experience loose stool or a mild bout of diarrhea. Reducing the intake usually solves the problem. I have routinely included 3,000 to 4,000 mg of vitamin C in my morning breakfast/vitamin routine. It may sound like a lot, mainly because we are conditioned to the "% Daily Value" we read on the "Nutrition Facts" panels on packaged foods. Incidentally, it only takes a miniscule 90 mg per day to achieve the "100% Daily Value" of vitamin C. So why take 3,000 mg? What most people do not realize is that those "Daily Value" percentages are just enough to avoid a deficiency.

If a person is already deficient in a certain nutrient, ingesting enough to reach 100% is not going to help the deficiency. These recommendations are, essentially, just enough to keep a person alive! Yet, in today's nutrient-draining, stress-filled world, most people are deficient in at least one nutrient or another. Thus, I think it is safe to say that meeting the "% Daily Value" of any particular nutrient is usually not enough. It's like trying to re-fill a quickly draining bathtub with a slowly dripping faucet.

Another simple nutrition fact that most of us miss is the sheer power of the nutrients in our food — as opposed to nutrients from a bottle. Nutrients that build our body must be in biochemical, life-producing form (remember, "life begets life"). Each of our organs tends to use one specific chemical element more than others and when we burn out the reserves held in our organs, symptoms arise that indicate deficiencies. When we get sick, it is an indication that we are low on one or more of these chemical elements. When we replace them, the body self-heals. One example of self-healing that most people grossly underestimate is the power afforded to the body through vitamin C (properly derived from a biochemical, life-producing form, not

> Vitamin C helps to heal bruises, wounds, fractures, and scar tissues. It strengthens blood vessels and supports a healthy appetite and stable moods.

a synthetic form). Vitamin C helps to heal bruises, wounds, fractures, and scar tissues. It strengthens blood vessels and supports a healthy appetite and stable moods. In fact, it supports overall good health including regular heartbeat, good digestion, and healthy levels of hemoglobin. Studies have also shown that Alzheimer's patients given anti-oxidants (in a formula containing vitamin C) demonstrate significantly improved cognitive scores.[14]

Research has also shown that people with higher vitamin C levels experienced 50% less death from cancer than those with low vitamin C levels. [15,16] Many of those with advanced lung[17] and colon cancers[18] who underwent intravenous vitamin C completely recovered, and as Dr. Thomas Levy mentions in his book *Primal Panacea* vitamin C has the potential to eradicate cancer altogether.

> Research has also shown that people with higher vitamin C levels experienced 50% less death from cancer than those with low vitamin C levels.

Ironically, as all-powerful as vitamin C may seem

to be, it is very fragile when exposed to heat. Some vitamins are affected by heat and others are not. Vitamin C is the most fragile in this respect. It is the first vitamin to be destroyed by heat. Keep that in mind when you buy over-the-counter cough and cold remedies. I'm from Canada, and in Canada we had a cough and cold remedy that came in a powder called "Neocitran". By the "citran" part of the name, one might assume that the mixture contained some measure of vitamin C, or at least some ascorbic acid.

It doesn't; it just tastes like citrus fruit. But even if it did, the effort to include vitamin C would be all for naught. This powder is similar to other cough and cold powders on the market in the USA; it is meant to be mixed with hot water and sipped as a soothing way to relieve symptoms so that you can sleep easier. Remember that vitamin C is the first vitamin to be affected by heat. If indeed the powder contained vitamin C and it was dropped into hot water, what would happen to the vitamin C? The heat of the hot water would destroy it.

Getting back to the cancer discussion for a moment, let's dream the impossible dream: What if there was a natural way to fight symptoms of two of the most common cancers in both women and men (breast cancer and prostate cancer, respectively). Better yet, what if there was a natural way to fight breast cancer and prostate cancer symptoms without side effects AND increase the effectiveness of conventional cancer treatments used in conjunction with natural healing techniques? The Creator of the universe is way ahead of us. Such a compound has always existed in the milk thistle plant: Silymarin.

I first learned about the power of silymarin in *The Blaylock Wellness Report*, written by Dr. Russell Blaylock, a nationally recognized board-certified neurosurgeon. Silymarin consists of flavonoids (silybin, isosilybin, silydianin and taxifoline) found in the milk thistle plant. Silymarin has long been heralded for its antioxidant and hepatoprotective (liver protective) qualities and is now being researched for its anticancer attributes in both breast and colon cancers. In breast cancer, it works by interfering with cancer growth. It binds to estrogen receptors, essentially putting up the "no vacancy" sign to cancer, preventing tumor growth[19] and, amazingly, goes exactly where it is needed, accumulating its cancer fighting power in breast tumor tissue.[20]

Equally remarkable, silymarin does something quite the opposite to help men deal with prostate cancer. Instead of "putting up the no vacancy sign", it opens a door. Aggressive types of prostate cancer are typically unresponsive to conventional radiation treatment, but silymarin helps by being a "radiosensitizing" agent; it opens the door of cancer cells, putting out the "welcome mat" for radiation therapy to do its thing far more effectively. In fact, one study in 2015 showed that use of silymarin in conjunction with radiation therapy resulted in a "10-fold higher apoptotic response" (i.e. 10 times better cancer cell kill rate). And get this: The silymarin only helped to kill the cancer cells and actually protected nearby normal cells that typically experience radiation poisoning and injury.[21]

> Vitamin E has been shown to reduce lung cancer risk by up to 53%.

Silymarin also beats cancer at its own game in the colon. As a survival mechanism, colon cancer cells will suppress their vitamin D receptors in an effort to protect themselves from vitamin D's cancer-fighting effects. Silymarin reverses the effect, allowing vitamin D to break into the cancer cells and do what it does best: stop the cells' proliferation and spread.[22]

Speaking of vitamins and cancer, vitamin E is another potent weapon. Most people dismiss vitamin E as a beauty supplement or an antioxidant, but it's so much more. Taking 300 IU of natural (not synthetic) vitamin E per day has been shown to reduce lung cancer risk by up to 53%.[23] Furthermore, research published in the *International Journal of Cancer* has shown that gamma-tocotrienol (a cofactor found

> This same vitamin E cofactor has also been shown to be effective against existing prostate tumors.

in natural vitamin E preparations) kills prostate cancer stem cells (cancer stem cells are the root of the disease from which cancer can recur).[24] This same vitamin E cofactor has also been shown to be effective against existing prostate tumors.[25,26]

As I'm sure you are beginning to see, each vitamin

has a specific role (indeed many specific roles) in the body. Thus, deficiencies in any vitamin can cause health problems. You could be deficient in several of them or just one. The same goes for every other nutrient in the body: Deficiencies cause problems.

# WHAT IS A MINERAL?

> Organic minerals come from plants; they are bioavailable. What that means is that they are very absorbable into the cells of the human body.

Like the official definition of a vitamin, the definition of a mineral is surprisingly simple. A mineral is "an organic substance needed by the human body for good health." Now let's stop for a minute and examine an important word in that definition: Organic. Typically, when we see this word, we are conditioned to think of organic vs conventional produce; in other words, grown without chemicals or genetically modified seeds. That is indeed one definition of organic, but that's not what we're talking about here. Organic in the sense of "organic minerals" means that the mineral was derived from something living. Organic minerals come from plants; they are bioavailable. What that means is that they are very absorbable into the cells of the human body. Organic minerals break down slowly, increasing their stability. This stability enables organic minerals to complete their journey to the parts of the body where they are needed without breaking away and binding to other compounds in the body, which would render them less absorbable or even completely unabsorbable.

Inorganic minerals, on the other hand, are mineral salts derived from non-living things (i.e. rocks and soil). Inorganic minerals are less bioavailable because they are less stable. They have a tendency to become "unbound" too quickly; they may bind with other molecules that make them less bioavailable or even completely unabsorbable. Obviously then, organic minerals are best to rebuild your cells, which are dying and being replaced at a rate of 300 million per minute (as you will recall from earlier in this book). So how do you know which type of mineral is being used in that supplement in your cupboard? Dr. Robert J. Thiel, author of *Naturopathy for the 21st Century* has a good rule of thumb:

"Most mineral salts are listed on the label with a two-word description, while most food complex minerals list the mineral and the source. For example, if next to the word 'calcium' the label says 'carbonate', it is clear that this is a mineral salt. If on the other hand, next to the word 'calcium' it says it is in a food complex (or otherwise states the food source) then it is usually from a food (it is of interest to note that calcium citrate is actually the rock known as limestone processed with lactic and citric acids — it is not a product of citrus fruits)." [27]

Incidentally, your body cannot convert inorganic minerals into organic minerals — only plants can do that. The plant's roots go into the soil, absorb the mineral salt, and convert it into something that is best for the human body to use. That's why plants are so important to human health.

Each mineral, whether organic or inorganic, is also classified as either a macro mineral or a trace mineral. A macro mineral is a mineral of which your body needs a relatively large amount. Macro minerals include calcium, magnesium, phosphorus, potassium, sulfur, chlorine, and sodium. A trace mineral is a mineral of which your body needs only a small amount. Trace minerals include iron, zinc, manganese, copper, molybdenum, iodine, chromium, and selenium.

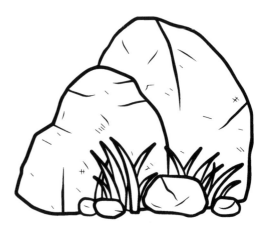

# WHY RAW FOOD?

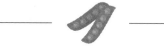

You may have heard that raw food is better for you in terms of all of these nutrients. Why is raw food hyped as being so much better than cooked food? Because raw food has enzymes — the life force of all living things — that, when ingested, transfer that life force to your body, helping it to repair and rebuild.

> When you give the body what it needs to build up its own defenses, your body can overcome almost anything.

Raw foods rebuild the body's self-healing ability so the body can reverse disease. When you give the body what it needs to build up its own defenses, your body can overcome almost anything.

During my five years as the senior staff writer with The Hallelujah Diet, I met hundreds of people who had empowered their immune systems by adopting a diet of primarily raw, plant-based food and overcame everything from seasonal allergies to diabetes, to heart disease, and even advanced-stage cancer. One widely known example of the power of the immune system is the story of Dr. Lorraine Day. She had breast cancer, but not just in her breast. She had a protruding tumor that looked like a tennis ball on her sternum. As part of her therapy, she had the bulk of the tumor removed, yet the cancer had already spread and progressed to the point that Dr. Day was on her deathbed. She couldn't move.

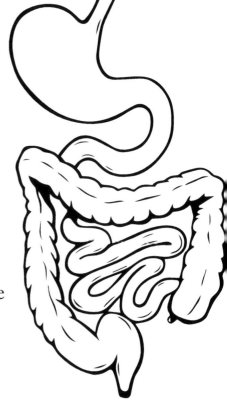

She couldn't even drink the raw carrot juice that people were making for her in an effort to empower her immune system — but there was another way. Instead of drinking the carrot juice, Dr. Day's care team administered raw vegetable juice enemas. That may seem awfully strange if you've never considered the colon as more than a waste stream, but the truth is that your colon is a crucial part of your body's nutrient absorption system. In fact, as a result of that "last ditch" effort to reverse the cancer, Dr. Day completely recovered.

Dr. Day's story serves as an example that the human body has amazing healing abilities if only provided with conditions conducive to do so. If a particular weak gene for one ailment or another runs in your family, you might have to be more careful about what you eat or what you do compared to your neighbor, but nutrition controls genetic expression. That means your food choices have the power to control whether that defective gene ever manifests its threat. The power to protect yourself and even reverse symptoms of disease is within you and the key to that "secret passage" is what you choose to eat.

> The power to protect yourself and even reverse symptoms of disease is within you and the key to that "secret passage" is what you choose to eat.

So what exactly is within raw foods that empowers the self-healing abilities of the human body?

Let's look at three of the main superstars inside raw foods: phytonutrients, antioxidants, and enzymes. Some of these terms, incidentally, can be attributed to both raw and cooked foods. Some antioxidants and phytonutrients, for example, are retained or even increased when they're cooked. For example, lycopene in tomatoes will actually increase with cooking. Other nutrients are lost in cooking, like vitamin C. However, we know that raw food contains phytonutrients, antioxidants, and enzymes so we are going to focus on raw foods for this discussion.

First, what is a phytonutrient? "Phyto" comes from the ancient Greek word phutón, meaning "plant". Thus a phytonutrient is defined as a plant substance that benefits health — a plant nutrient. By definition, foods like meat, cheese, eggs, and all other animal-derived foods do not have phytonutrients; you will never find a phytonutrient in an animal-derived food. Phytonutrients are kind of an ambiguous thing. They're not a vitamin or a mineral. There are over 10,000 kinds. There are phytonutrients that are antioxidant in nature, anti-inflammatory, antiviral, and antibacterial.

Phytonutrients are most abundant in brightly colored fruits and vegetables. This is part of the genius of the Almighty's creation. He created humans to see color. We see a colorful fruit or vegetable and instinctively reach for it as something that looks good to eat.

For example, beta carotene (a phytonutrient) is the bright orange pigment that you see in carrots that the human liver converts into vitamin A. Lycopene (a phytonutrient) is the pigment that makes tomatoes and watermelon appear red. Other phytonutrients include flavonoids in berries and sulforaphane in broccoli; when broccoli is on the verge of going bad, the sulphur scent you smell comes from the phytonutrient sulforaphane. Sulforaphane is found in especially high concentrations in broccoli sprouts.

Incidentally, sulforaphane is now being investigated as a protectant against sun damage to the skin. It's not a sunscreen per se, but boosts the protection of certain enzymes in the human body to protect skin against UV damage from the inside out. In fact, researchers at Johns Hopkins University found that sulforaphane, when applied topically, provided effective protection against UV radiation damage and thus potentially against skin cancer.

The study noted that increasing the body's own cell-protective mechanisms (through topical application of sulforaphane) "protects against damage of a carcinogen that is ubiquitous in our environment and represents the principal etiological factor for the development of human skin cancers."[28] In a press release, research authors went into further detail, noting the powerful effects of the extract:

"At the highest doses, UV-induced redness and inflammation were reduced by an average of 37%. The [sulforaphane] extracts were protective even when applied three days prior to UV exposure. The protection did vary considerably among the subjects, ranging from 8% to 78%, which [the research author] notes may be due to genetic differences among individuals, local differences in the skin, or other factors such as dietary habits. He also points out that conventional sunscreens were essentially ineffective in these experiments."

This example demonstrates how the human body's cell-protective mechanisms can be increased by eating foods that contain phytonutrients. It's what a person eats that prepares the body to deal with the sun, because everything we eat is fuel for our organs. And skin is the human body's largest organ. Just like the brain, kidneys, spleen, or liver, skin is an organ. We need to provide our skin with nutrients from the food we eat so that when the skin is exposed to sunlight, it is prepared to protect itself from the inside out like an internal sunscreen, if you will.

> Did you know that sunscreen not only blocks UV rays but also blocks your body's vitamin D production?

Speaking of sunscreen, did you know that sunscreen not only blocks UV rays but also blocks your body's vitamin D production? For example, if you put on sunscreen before going out in the sun, you won't get any vitamin D. My family and I have a different strategy. When we go to the beach, we don't put on sunscreen right away. We spend about

20 to 30 minutes in the sun first (or less on the first beach trip of the year when our skin has been indoors for months and is more likely to burn), then we put on sunscreen, lightweight, breathable sun-protective clothing, or a combination of both.

Let's get into our next raw food substance: Antioxidants. What is an antioxidant? Quite simply, it is a substance that inhibits oxidation. Oxidation is the action that makes iron patio furniture rusty when it's left out in the rain. Why does it get rusty? First, the water combines with carbon dioxide in the air to form a weak carbonic acid that begins to dissolve the iron. Then the water will begin to break down into hydrogen and oxygen. The free oxygen binds with the iron and changes the molecular structure of the iron. The same thing happens inside your body's cells.

Think of oxidation like a campfire. It's a fire created by your body's metabolism that produces toxins in your body. Any time your body burns calories, you are creating that campfire; you are oxidizing. In fact, the

word, 'calorie' is a measure of heat. And just like
the heat, smoke, and resulting ash of a campfire,
metabolism also produces toxins and ash (make a
mental note of the word "ash", we'll come back to it
in a minute). In the body, metabolic toxins become
free radicals — unpaired electrons that cause a
damage domino effect in your body. We talked about
this earlier in the first section of this book:

"A free radical is a molecule that lacks an electron,
making it unstable and damaging to the body as it
hunts for an electron to "rob" from another molecule
in order to regain its stability. Every time a molecule
is robbed of an electron, it causes cellular damage.
Alternatively, every antioxidant contains an extra
electron in its molecular structure with the express
purpose of "donating" that extra electron to a free
radical molecule in order to stabilize the free radical,
thereby halting its damaging behavior."

Excess free radicals cause cellular damage, as you
can imagine. And cellular damage leads to disease.
Antioxidants prevent that damage because they have
extra electrons.

Now, with that in mind, let's get back to the word

"ash". When your body metabolizes ("burns") food, just like a campfire, you are left with ash. Depending on the type of food consumed, that ash will be either acidic or alkaline. Plant foods leave your body with alkaline ash. That's a good thing. Animal-derived foods and processed foods leave an acid ash. That's bad; acidity leads to disease. As a general rule, alkaline ash-forming foods are those foods that are GROWN IN the ground; acid ash-forming foods are those that WALK ON the ground. It's a little more complicated than that, but generally, if the food you are about to eat had a mother or a face, or if it was processed, think twice.

The terms "acid" and "alkaline" are determined by the pH (potential hydrogen) scale, measured from 0 to 14. Zero is extreme acid. Fourteen is extreme alkaline. As you might imagine, water is typically right in the middle, neutral, at seven. Anything below seven is acid. Anything above seven is alkaline. Human blood is 7.38 – 7.44 on the alkaline side. Naturally, you would assume your body would be most in harmony with foods that leave an alkaline ash — and your assumption would be correct.

When you eat something that leaves an acidic ash,

your body is thrown into battle. It must maintain its alkalinity or die. Anything that causes acidity pressures the body to fight its way back to the alkaline side of the scale. This fight is what causes oxidative stress, which leads to free radicals, and the disease domino effect begins.

> When you eat acidic foods such as meat, cheese, dairy, processed foods, what happens? Among other maladies, the acid/alkaline battle will weaken bones.

How does your body fight its way back to alkalinity? It must find something alkaline within itself to neutralize the acid. And what is one of the most alkaline substances in the human body? Calcium — in your bones, specifically. So here's what happens: When threatened with acidity, the body uses every available source of alkalinity it has to neutralize the disease-causing, acid threat. It does this by pulling calcium from the bones, leading to bone porosity, weakness, and calcified arteries.

When you eat acidic foods such as meat, cheese, dairy, processed foods, what happens? Among other maladies, the acid/alkaline battle will weaken bones. But "what about milk, cheese, and yogurt?" you may ask. "These foods come from animal, yet they are touted as having a lot of calcium, which is good for the bones." That statement is true, but those who promote that message are not telling the whole story.

Yes, calcium is indeed good for the bones. However, the acid-forming nature of dairy forces the human body into the acid/alkaline battle, during which it uses every bit of calcium in the dairy to neutralize the dairy's acidic effects — the problem is, it's not enough. The acid-forming nature of the dairy is greater than its inherent amount of alkaline-forming calcium can handle. So, to make up the difference, the body is required to pull additional calcium from the bones to completely neutralize the acid-forming threat.

Now, let's stop and think about this for a moment. If the body of the person who consumes dairy is forced to use all of the calcium in the dairy in an attempt to neutralize the acid-forming nature of the dairy, PLUS pull calcium from its own bones to completely neutralize the acid threat, did the dairy really "give" that person ANY calcium? No. In fact, that person is left with LESS calcium than they had before consuming the dairy. That's right. Consuming dairy actually results in NEGATIVE net calcium.

So, where do you get your calcium? As a general rule, green and orange foods are great sources of calcium, like romaine lettuce, kale (arguably the best source of calcium), broccoli, carrot juice, sweet potato, almonds, and tahini (made with sesame seeds; tahini is a common ingredient in hummus). These foods are great because they also have healthy levels of magnesium, which is necessary to offset the calcium. Dairy has massive amounts of calcium but hardly any magnesium, which causes an imbalance.

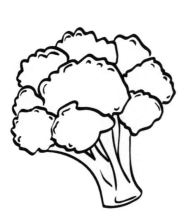 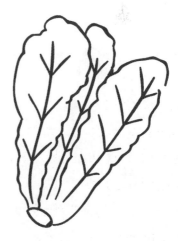

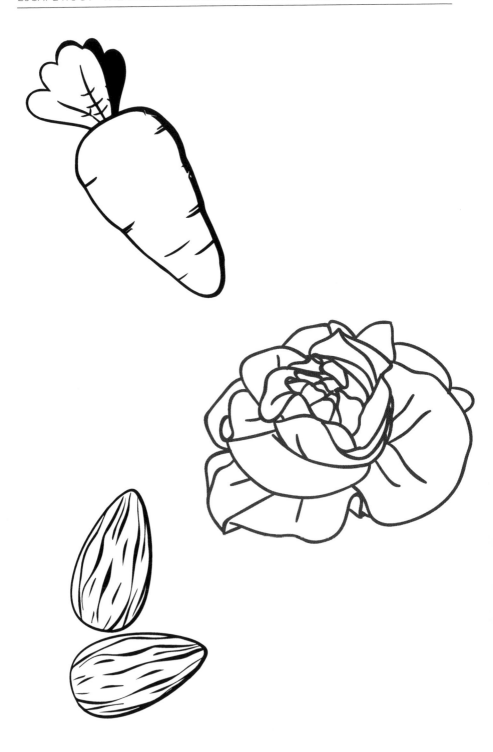

# WHAT IS AN ENZYME?

An enzyme is an energized protein molecule that exists in every cell that initiates chemical reactions. Our body depends on chemical reactions to see, hear, think, breathe, and perform practically every function it is capable of. Enzymes also facilitate digestion and the utilization of nutrients.

> To see if a packaged item contains enzymes, look for "-ase" at the end of the word. Serrapeptase, for example.

There are three types of enzymes: Metabolic enzymes, digestive enzymes and food enzymes. Here's an enzyme identification exercise you can do the next time you're at the grocery store or health food store: To see if a packaged item contains enzymes, look for "-ase" at the end of the word. Serrapeptase, for example, is a supplement that I use quite frequently. It is a proteolytic enzyme, which means it "seeks and destroys" excess proteins. In plain language, this means it "eats" inflammation and undigested proteins such as blood clots, scar tissue, cysts, mucus, arterial plaque, and inflammation in all forms without

> Metabolic enzymes are enzymes that promote energy production, detoxification, and cell repair.

any harmful side effects. It is the same enzyme the silkworm uses to dissolve its cocoon, which is a protein. Whenever one of our family members has a bump or a bruise or inflammation from an accident, the first thing we do is give them serrapeptase; the inflammation subsides in a fraction of the time and it gives their body a head-start on healing. If you decide to try it, just remember that serrapeptase must be taken on an empty stomach; if there's food in your stomach, serrapeptase's protein-eating action will be wasted on digesting your food instead of seeking out undigested proteins elsewhere in your body.

Now, back to our definitions. Metabolic enzymes are enzymes that promote energy production, detoxification, and cell repair. Digestive enzymes break down food; they are created in the pancreas. Food enzymes are found in raw foods. Each raw food has its own enzymes that ripen, break down and digest that particular food. When you eat an apple, for example, the Almighty has created the enzymes in that apple to specifically break down that apple in your digestive system so that you don't have to use your own digestive enzymes (from your pancreas). This is the beauty of raw food — it helps to digest itself. The opposite is true of cooked or processed food. Cooking and processing destroys the enzymes that would have helped to digest the raw food (enzymes are destroyed by heat above 122°F). With all naturally-occurring food enzymes destroyed, all of the work of digesting cooked or processed food is now completely dependent on your own enzymes produced in your pancreas. This is the danger of too much cooked food. It stresses the organs. You probably eat more cooked food than you think.

Enzymes begin to die at around 108°F and are completely dead at 122°F. Now, think about this —

water boils at 212°F. However, some people claim that if they steam broccoli, it is still alive. Well, how hot is that steam? It's the same temperature as the boiling water, so even steaming food will destroy enzymes. If the food is hot, the enzymes are dead.

Here's another surprising fact: The life force of enzymes can be seen on photographic film using a process called Kirlian photography. The process was developed in 1939 by Russian inventor and researcher Semyon Kirlian but wasn't widely recognized until the 1960s. Kirlian photography is like an x-ray that reveals the life force (enzymes) in raw food. They show up on photographic film like bright white stars on a clear night. For example, if an apple is cut in half and laid flat on photographic film, then the film is charged with high voltage, the resulting image shows the apple with evenly distributed, equally bright "stars" throughout the flesh of the apple. If the apple is cooked or denatured in any way, the image shows vast areas of darkness interspersed with random, disjointed clusters of light in varying intensities — clearly different than the naturally-occurring, orderly nature of the original enzymatic life force of the raw apple. Now, think back to phrases you've heard in the

Bible: "I am the light" and "I am the life." The Messiah describes himself as life and light. The life in that apple is literally light, which should not be surprising when one considers that everything on this earth depends on light from the sun. Raw, living plant foods store this light energy as biophotons, the smallest physical units of light. Biophotons are stored in and used by both raw, living, plant-based foods and by the human body, and may play a significant part of our body's biochemical reactions. Much of this science is still being investigated, but it appears that foods that store the most "light" (i.e. biophotons) are most nutritious. These biophotons are then transferred to the human body when raw foods are consumed, affording more energy to the body for healing. Amazing!

Do you see how nature clearly connects to the Almighty and his Word? It's no wonder that eating raw foods that grow from the ground was His first and foremost plan for the life and health of mankind (Genesis 1:29). On a personal note, it seems obvious to me that the Almighty gave the idea of Kirlian photography to Mr. Kirlian in order to reveal Himself — light and life — in that raw apple.

If light and life are found in enzymatically-alive foods, is the opposite true of foods devoid of living enzymes? Indeed, without food enzymes to help digestion, cooked or processed food will overtax the pancreas. In turn, an overtaxed pancreas will summon help from the immune system, a function called digestive leukocytosis. The term leukocytosis refers to an increase in white blood cells, indicating the body is in attack mode; this commonly occurs when you are sick. This is how cooked food can break down the immune system. You may have noticed that, after eating a large portion of cooked food at a family meal or party, you feel under the weather the next day, maybe even like you "caught a cold," or you feel achy and have a headache (even if no alcohol was consumed). This is the body reacting to too much cooked food; it taxed your pancreas and, in turn, your immune system. Over time, a perpetually taxed pancreas and immune system can spell disaster for your health as your body is starved of the light and life it needs to survive.

# WHERE DO YOU GET YOUR PROTEIN?

Protein is commonly referred to as the biological building block of life. Protein is made of amino acids; there are 22 standard amino acids, nine of which are essential. You will remember from the vitamin section of this book that the word "essential" means that the body cannot make the nutrient autonomously. It must be derived from food. Foods with sufficient levels of all nine essential amino acids are called "complete" proteins.

What about protein combining? Frances Moore Lappé developed this theory in the 1970s, which claimed that all nine essential amino acids were required to be consumed in the same meal, otherwise the body would not benefit from a complete protein. Ten years later, after much research, she dismissed her own theory. Indeed, foods do not need to be combined to make a complete protein because proteins are broken down into amino acids once you eat them. If one or more of the essential amino acids to make a complete protein is missing, the body simply waits until the missing pieces are available, then reassembles the amino acid puzzle to make a complete protein and distributes it to the body as needed. Surprisingly, though the theory of protein combining has been dismissed for decades (by its own developer, no less), somehow it is still validated by some.

What about getting protein from plants? Is that even possible? Consider a typical laundry stain-remover commercial that claims to remove "protein stains" — like blood and grass. Have you ever heard a commercial like that? If there's no protein in a plant (i.e. grass), why would they use it as an example of a "protein" stain? In fact, you may recall that enzymes are "energized protein molecules". Therefore, every living plant food has protein.

You may have also heard the terms "high quality" and "low quality" protein. These terms are a bit of a misnomer; one is not "better" than the other (in fact, in terms of overall health, the opposite is true). Simply defined, the term high quality protein refers to a food that contains sufficient levels of all nine essential amino acids so as to be considered a "complete" protein. The term low quality protein refers to a food that is missing sufficient levels of one or more of the nine essential amino acids and is thus considered an "incomplete" protein. However, this does NOT mean that a "low quality" protein is inferior. It simply means that the particular food in question does not have sufficient levels of ALL nine essential amino acids. Remember what you just read about protein combining: Having all nine essential amino acids in one sitting is not necessary; your body breaks down and reassembles amino acids to create complete protein anyway. So, as long as you consume a variety of "low quality" protein foods containing sufficient levels of all nine amino acids within the variety of said foods, you are indeed consuming "complete protein". And that's OK.

In fact, it's better than OK. The human body likes to keep stress low, but metabolizing a complete protein all at once (i.e. meat) is stressful. The human body prefers the steady, gentle, ebb and flow of metabolizing plant foods, which makes sense considering that a plant-based diet was the Almighty's original intent for mankind. Breaking down and reassembling protein from a plant-based diet with a few essential amino acids here and a few more there is the way the human body likes to do things.

Our bodies are designed for plant foods. Let's compare the human body to the body of a dog, which is made to eat meat, starting with the jaw. A human jaw is made to move up and down, side to side, which is perfect for grinding food but is not great for tearing flesh. A dog's jaw and teeth are designed to tear flesh and crush bone. The acid of a dog's stomach is also stronger than a human's, which means a dog is able to break down meat more efficiently than a human can. Finally, and most importantly, a dog's intestines are shorter than a human's. The waste from meat is expelled from a dog's body in a much shorter time period than that of human's body. And that's the key. With all the bends and twists in the human digestive tract, meat spends far too much time in the 98.6° Fahrenheit environment of the human body. Here's a hypothesis that was related

> Meat rots in the intestines because it simply takes too long to make its way through.

to me by the founder of The Hallelujah Diet, Rev. George Malkmus: Imagine leaving meat on your kitchen counter, then turning up the heat to 98° Fahrenheit and leaving the house for three days. When you came back to the house, that meat would be rotten! That's exactly what happens to the meat a person consumes; it rots in the intestines because it simply takes too long to make its way through. Not to mention, rotting flesh will produce carcinogens when fed with pathogenic bacteria in the human gut. Plant foods, on the other hand, are what the human body is designed for. The waste is expelled quickly because the protein is much easier for the human body to break down and utilize.

Now, how much protein do you need? Probably much less than you think! Here's a simple calculation: Take your weight in pounds and divide by 2.2. This will give you your weight in kilograms (we do this because we want to talk about protein in terms of grams, which is metric). Now, multiply your weight in kilograms by 0.8. This is your recommended protein intake.

For example, a 150-lb person needs 54.5 grams of protein per day ([150 lbs. / 2.2] x 0.8 = 54.5). That is what you need to maintain a healthy diet. People ask, "how am I ever going to get 54.5 grams if I'm eating just plant food?"

Guess what? One cup of cooked lentils — a mere side dish — contains 18 grams of protein. You're a third of the way there already, in ONE side dish! It's easy. Very easy. You'll eat things during the day you don't even know have protein, because every living food that has enzymes has protein. You're giving your body little bits at a time. People on a plant-based diet rarely have difficulty getting enough protein.

**People on a plant-based diet rarely have difficulty getting enough protein.**

To meet recommended intakes of protein, it is important to include higher protein selections of vegetables, beans, nuts, seeds, and grains. The calories from protein in most green vegetables and legumes range from 20% to 40% and in nuts and seeds from 9% to 17%. At the low end of the spectrum is fruit, with just 2% to 10% of the calories from protein.

In short, a plant-based diet provides more than enough protein. In fact, the concern of "getting enough" protein should really be a concern of getting too much! Abundant research has shown that a diet of 20% (animal) protein or more promotes cancer growth.[23] A diet of 10% protein is considered optimal (even for children and bodybuilders), but only 5-6% protein is actually needed to replace the protein your body uses.

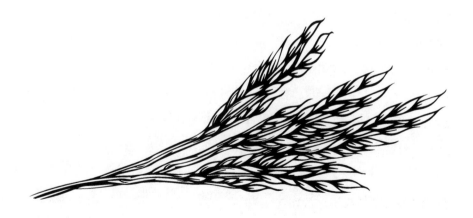

## Protein Content of Selected Plant-Based Foods

| Food | Serving | Protein (g) | Protein (g/100 cal) |
| --- | --- | --- | --- |
| Lentils, cooked | 1 cup | 18 | 7.8 |
| Black beans, cooked | 1 cup | 15 | 6.7 |
| Kidney beans, cooked | 1 cup | 13 | 6.4 |
| Chickpeas, cooked | 1 cup | 12 | 4.2 |
| Baked beans | 1 cup | 12 | 5.0 |
| Pinto beans, cooked | 1 cup | 12 | 5.7 |
| Black-eyed peas, cooked | 1 cup | 11 | 6.2 |
| Lima beans, cooked | 1 cup | 10 | 5.7 |
| Quinoa, cooked | 1 cup | 9 | 3.5 |
| Peas, cooked | 1 cup | 9 | 6.4 |
| Spaghetti, cooked | 1 cup | 8 | 3.7 |
| Almonds | 1/4 cup | 8 | 3.7 |
| Bulgur wheat, cooked | 1 cup | 6 | 3.7 |
| Sunflower seeds | 1/4 cup | 6 | 3.3 |
| Cashews | 1/4 cup | 5 | 2.7 |
| Almond butter | 2 Tbsp | 5 | 2.4 |
| Brown rice, cooked | 1 cup | 5 | 2.1 |
| Broccoli | 1 cup | 4 | 6.8 |
| Potato, baked | 1 med.(6 oz) | 4 | 2.7 |

To meet recommended intakes of protein the important question is not, "Where do you get your protein?" The better question to ask is, "Where do you get your carbohydrates?" That's what really matters.

# WHERE DO YOU GET YOUR CARBOHYDRATES?

What are carbohydrates? Carbohydrates are sugars, starches, and cellulose that provide energy to the body. Not all carbohydrates are the same, however, so don't get caught by the myth that "all carbs are bad". That's not right. There are two types of carbohydrates and how they react in the body is vastly different.

Simple carbs in processed and refined foods like breads and candy equal simple sugar, they digest very quickly. Quickly digesting sugar delivers a punch to the body — too much, too fast. A sucker punch is a more accurate description. Even in their chemical structure, simple carbohydrates are literally "simple"; there's not much to them, so the body doesn't have to work very hard to break the structure apart. Fast digestion, as we get with simple carbs, equals a high glycemic index. You don't want this.

Complex carbohydrates, on the other hand, digest slower; these are the carbohydrates found in whole, plant-based foods. They digest slower and are therefore more in harmony with the ebb and flow of the body's processes, as discussed in the protein section of this book. Your body runs on complex carbohydrates. You can't live without them.

Simply put, changing the quality of your carbohydrates can change the quality of your health and life. And while you may not be able to avoid all simple carbs (i.e. sugars), it's best to be informed on which sugars (or alternative sweeteners) pose the least amount of threat to your health. Limit your consumption of sugars overall and avoid processed foods to the best of your ability. Sugar and many other health-prohibiting ingredients are almost always found in processed foods. Make sure you can read and UNDERSTAND the label. After all, what you don't know CAN hurt you.

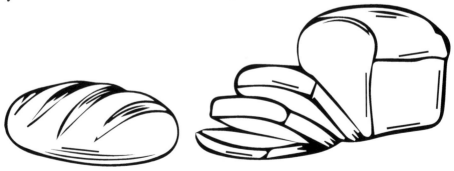

# WHERE DO YOU GET YOUR FIBER?

Speaking of whole, plant-based foods, let's get into dietary fiber for a moment. Here again there are two kinds: Soluble and insoluble. Soluble fiber will dissolve in water; this is the type of fiber that makes you feel full. Insoluble fiber does not dissolve in water. The job of insoluble fiber is to speed waste away. It helps get the toxins out of your body. Incidentally, efficient toxin flow is extremely important for good health. This means that you should be having a bowel movement every day, at least, not every second day or every three days. I'm going to sound like Dr. Oz here for a second, but you want feces that look like a snake.

> The job of insoluble fiber is to speed waste away. It helps get the toxins out of your body.

Soft, abundant, and not hard to pass. If you have a movement like this every day, you know you're doing most things right.

Eating large quantities of food rich in fiber is going to be the primary means of helping your body to collect and speed away waste. The best foods in this category are green foods — specifically dark, leafy greens. Why? Leafy greens are loaded with chlorophyll. In fact, chlorophyll is what gives greens their color. And what's really amazing about chlorophyll is that, under a microscope, it looks a lot like hemoglobin, a protein in your blood that transports oxygen throughout your body.

Both hemoglobin and chlorophyll have a ring in their molecular structure. In the case of chlorophyll, this ring does an excellent job of binding to carcinogens in your gut and ushering them out of the body, preventing them from damaging your vital organs. Essentially, chlorophyll is a chelator (the word "chelate" was originally used in 1826 as a zoology term to describe an animal with claws.) The word "chelation", in chemical terms, is the molecular equivalent of grasping and pulling away. That's

Soluble fiber is found in oatmeal, oat cereal, apples, lentils, oranges, pears, oat bran, strawberries, nuts, flaxseeds, beans, peas, cucumbers, celery, carrots, and so on.

why green plants are so good for you. The chlorophyll in them is a chelator; it literally pulls away and disposes of toxins, protecting you from the domino effect of free radical activity, inflammation, and disease. So, obviously you want to eat a lot of chlorophyll-rich foods in your diet, and eating raw, leafy greens and other whole (not processed), plant-based foods rich in fiber is an easy way to do that.

Both soluble and insoluble fiber are important for good digestion, heart health, weight management, bowel function, etc. So where do we get fiber? This is easy. Soluble fiber is found in oatmeal, oat cereal, apples, lentils, oranges, pears, oat bran, strawberries, nuts, flaxseeds, beans, peas, cucumbers, celery, carrots, and so on.

Sources of insoluble fiber are found in the same types of foods: Dark leafy vegetables, raisins, grapes, fruit, root vegetable skins, whole grains, seeds, nuts, barley, couscous, brown rice, zucchini, celery, broccoli, cabbage, onions, tomatoes, carrots, cucumbers, green beans, etc. Remember, there is not one ounce of fiber in any animal-derived food.

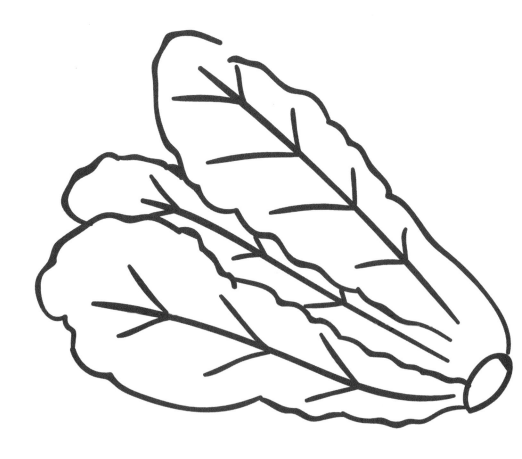

# WHERE DO YOU GET YOUR CALCIUM?

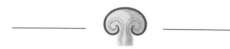

If you've already decided to change your lifestyle based on what you've read so far in this book, be prepared for questions about lack of nutrients from people who don't know any better. One of the most popular questions (other than "where do you get your protein?") is going to be: "Where do you get your calcium?" First, you want to make sure you're getting your calcium from living sources, not rocks (remember our "organic vs inorganic" discussion earlier). Most of the calcium supplements on store shelves come from rocks. Eat a well-rounded source of vegetable foods and you won't need those calcium supplements.

I received a good rule of thumb from a doctor I interviewed for my TV health show (*The Health Awakening*) in 2017. Her name is Dr. Carolyn Dean and she is an expert on dietary minerals, especially magnesium. Your body needs both magnesium and calcium to balance each other out. For example, muscles need calcium to contract, but they need magnesium in order to relax. An overabundance of calcium and not enough magnesium can spell disaster for your most important and most continually active muscle — your heart. Here is what she told me about the difference between these two minerals:

"Get your calcium from food, get your magnesium through supplementation. The U.K. and the World Health Organization both recommend about 600mg of calcium per day, and you can usually get that in your diet — deep green leafy vegetables, nuts and seeds, and so on. But because of conditions in the soil our food grows in, we need to get magnesium through supplementation. Therapeutic amounts of magnesium (through supplementation), by the way, will actually dissolve calcium that is built up in the wrong places in the body (arteries, kidneys), and directs it to where it belongs, in your bones."

If I was concerned about low calcium intake and wanted to boost it the right way (via food, not supplementation), I would try tahini. Tahini is like a peanut butter made with sesame seeds. It's common in many Mediterranean and Middle Eastern dishes and is also a main ingredient in hummus. Per gram, tahini contains almost triple the calcium of milk without the acidity that dairy causes. Other good sources of calcium include kale, romaine, and any other dark green leafy vegetable. Carrot juice, almonds, and sweet potatoes are all also good sources.

In fact, almost any orange or green plant-based food is going to have a good supply of calcium in a form your body can utilize. It's not the same story with animal-based foods. Remember from our "acid/alkaline" discussion in the "Why Raw Food?" section of this book that animal sources of calcium take more calcium than they give because of the inherent acidity they bring to the body.

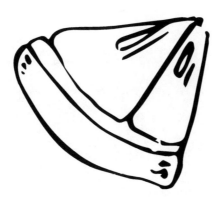

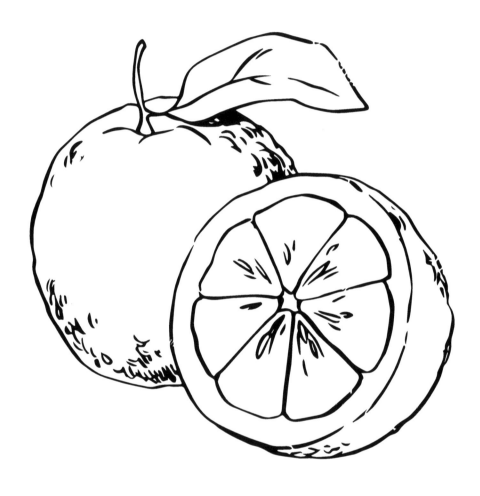

# WHAT ABOUT FAT?

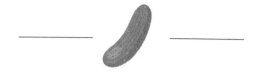

We all know there are good fats and bad fats. Fats are solidified animal or vegetable oil. If it's liquid, it's oil. If it's solid, it's fat. It's the same thing. Fat is a far more concentrated source of energy than protein or carbohydrates. Each gram of fat has 9 calories; protein and carbs each have 4 calories per gram. So there's more than double the amount of energy in fat, but there's a lot to know when it comes to fat, saturated or unsaturated. Short, medium, long chain fatty acids. Omega 3, 6 and 9. What does it all mean?

First, saturated fats are solid at room temperature, like coconut oil. You may have noticed in your pantry that, in winter, coconut oil is solid and in summer it is liquid. Unsaturated fats are liquid at room temperature; they also go rancid faster due to their molecular structure. Here's why: The molecular structure of any fat includes opportunities for hydrogen to bond with carbon. If all of these opportunities are occupied with hydrogen atoms, the fat is said to be "saturated" (i.e. saturated with hydrogen). If there are opportunities within the molecular structure that hydrogen has not occupied, the fat is said to be "unsaturated". A fat with one open opportunity in such a molecular structure is called "mono-unsaturated". A fat with two or more open opportunities for hydrogen in its molecular structure is called "polyunsaturated".

The open opportunities for hydrogen in the molecular structure of unsaturated fats can also be occupied by oxygen. When this happens, the fat is said to have become oxidized or rancid. The greater the number of open opportunities for oxygen to move into the molecular structure, the more susceptible the oil is to rancidity. This is why polyunsaturated fat (the type of fat with two or more open opportunities for hydrogen or oxygen) is at greatest risk for rancidity, followed by monounsaturated fat (having only one open opportunity for hydrogen or oxygen). Saturated fat is, logically, the most stable fat and most resistant to rancidity.

Now that you understand the role of hydrogen in fat, you have the basis to understand what "hydrogenated" oil is (the unnatural fat used to make many manufactured foods). Stable, saturated fat is ideal to make manufactured foods last longer, but other aspects of natural, saturated fats may be undesirable for manufacturing (cost, gumming up machines, etc.).

So, manufacturers select a more suitable, unsaturated fat for their purposes and "force" it to behave like a saturated fat. The result of such a process is a "hydrogenated" or "partially hydrogenated" oil. To hydrogenate an oil, manufacturers force hydrogen gas into liquid monounsaturated or polyunsaturated oil. The hydrogen then fills the gaps in the molecular structure, creating a more shelf-stable (artificially saturated) fat — albeit, a molecular structure not found in nature, which confuses and damages the human body when ingested.

Another term you may have heard regarding fats is "chain", as in short, medium, and long chain fatty acids. Fatty acid molecules literally look like a chain. Now, imagine a chain being pulled through a hole.

How much effort does it take to pull a short or medium size chain? Not very much. A long chain takes a lot of effort. That's how your body reacts to each different type of "chain" of fatty acid. The longer the chain, the more energy (and stress) it takes for your body to break down.

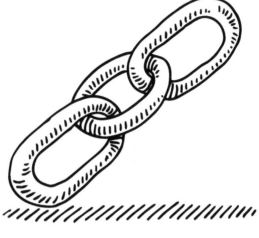

Short-chain fatty acids are produced in small amounts when dietary fiber (from plant-based food) is fermented in the colon. Medium chain fatty acids are fats that are burned for energy; they do not get stored as fat. Coconuts are one of the rare sources of medium chain fatty acids. The coconut's medium chain fatty acids are smaller than long-chain fatty acids, so they are more easily digested and they are converted to energy instead of being stored as fat. This type of antiviral, antimicrobial fat (42% to 57% lauric acid) is also found in human breast milk and can boost metabolism and weight loss. In a coconut oil research paper written for the Hallelujah Acres Foundation, Research Director Dr. Michael Donaldson notes, "There are only a very few good sources of lauric acid in nature—coconut oil (44-49%), palm kernel oil (~47%), and breast milk (4-10%, depending on diet). The lauric acid in breast milk, and the monolaurin formed in the baby's stomach, helps protect the baby from disease. This protection can be increased if the mother consumes coconut."

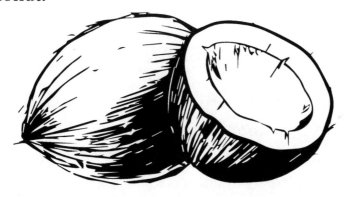

Another study involving tropical island inhabitants was conducted from the 1960s until 1981 to examine the relative effects of saturated fat and dietary cholesterol due to a diet that consisted mainly of coconuts (whose fat content is highly saturated). To the researchers' surprise, vascular disease was uncommon in both populations. This fact, along with others, led the researchers to conclude that "there is no evidence of the high saturated fat intake having a harmful effect."[30]

Now, this may be due to the fact that these populations consume coconut in its whole form, taking advantage of all of the nutrients in the food working in synergy together, combined with other tropical island lifestyle factors that not everyone can take advantage of. Fats should, ideally, be consumed in their natural state as part of a whole, plant-based food, not extracted as an oil alone (i.e. eating coconuts rather than consuming just the oil).

As a general rule for good health, consumption of any extracted oils should be significantly limited (or even eliminated) in any form, saturated or unsaturated. Getting back to our "chain" discussion, some long chain fatty acids are healthy, while others are not, depending on sum total qualities of the fat. The long chain fatty acids in saturated animal fats, for example, are something you want to avoid. (Are you starting to see a pattern, here? Once again, animal-derived foods are not ideal for human health.)

In fact, according to a press release on the website for the Physicians Committee for Responsible Medicine:

"Women following vegan diets have significantly more omega-3 (long chain) 'good fats' in their blood, compared with fish-eaters, meat-eaters, and ovo-lacto vegetarians, according to a new report from the European Prospective Investigation into Cancer and Nutrition (EPIC) Study. Levels in vegan men were not quite as high as in vegan women. Despite zero intake of long-chain omega-3s, eicosapentaenoic acid (EPA) and docosahexaenoic acid (DHA), and substantially lower intake of their plant-derived precursor alpha-linolenic acid (ALA), vegan participants converted robust amounts of shorter-chain fatty acids into these long-chain fatty acids."[31]

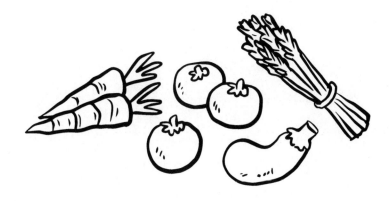

Very briefly, here is a rule of thumb I use to explain the difference between omega 3, 6, and 9 fatty acids:

- **"Omega-3, more please."** That's what your body is saying; these are the helpful types of essential fatty acids. Our food supply is such that getting "too many" omega 3 fatty acids compared to omega 6 is highly unlikely. Plant-based foods highest in omega-3 fatty acids include flaxseeds, walnuts, and chia seeds.

- **"Too much omega-6 can make you sick."** The Physicians Committee for Responsible Medicine website says it best: "Omega-6 fatty acids compete with omega-3 fatty acids for use in the body, and therefore excessive intake of omega-6 fatty acids (from processed foods and extracted oils) can inhibit omega-3s. Ideally, the ratio of omega-6 to omega-3 fatty acids should be between 1:1 and 4:1. Instead, most Americans consume these fatty acids at a ratio of 10:1 and 25:1 and are consequently unable to reap the benefits of omega-3s."[32, 33, 34] Omega-6 essential fatty acids are found mostly in oils, which are used often in processed foods."

- **"Omega-9 is just fine."** Omega 9s are non-essential fats, which means that your body creates them on its own. If you give it more through healthy fats, that's just fine. Again, these fats should come from plant source foods like sunflower seeds, hazelnuts, macadamia nuts, and almond butter.

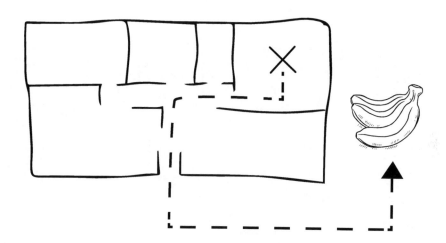

# PART 3

## EXECUTING YOUR ESCAPE PLAN

# THE LAWS OF HEALTH

In chapter 25 of one of my favorite health books, *The Chemistry of Man*, author Bernard Jensen lists what he considers to be the "fundamental laws of health". As a preamble to these laws, he states, "We must return to God and nature; this is a return to our true self. Nature does the curing; all it needs is an opportunity." To accomplish this, Jensen urges the reader to understand axioms and principles for proper nutrition and good health — his "laws of health" — including:[35]

- The chemical elements that build our body must be in biochemical, life-producing form. They must come to us as food, magnetically, electrically alive, grown from the dust of the earth.

- Healthy plant life requires all the chemical elements in the proper, balanced order.

- The animal that lives on plant life (including humans) molds to the food it eats.

- Our body is a storehouse for the chemical elements. Each organ tends to use one specific chemical element more than others according to the law of balance and proportion.

- With a knowledge of the workings of the chemical elements within the body, we can look at a person and tell immediately when he lacks certain chemical elements. When we burn out the specific chemical reserves held in our organs, we produce symptoms that indicate these deficiencies.

- Whenever we are sick, we are short of at least one chemical element. We must pay back what we "owe" the body. When we take in these chemical elements, health returns.

- Every symptom is a sign of a chemical shortage in the body. When you feel sick or even look sick, you are lacking in one or more chemical elements.

- When regaining health, you don't take "two tablespoons" of some remedy and get immediately well; however, you're on the way to getting well the minute you begin filling the body with the missing chemical elements.

- Because "two tablespoons" are good for you, that doesn't mean "four tablespoons" are even better. Nature builds one drop at a time. You take two tablespoons every day for six months; that's how you get well.

- We are like a plant. We can get well, but we must have the right nutrients and other conditions to grow and thrive. We have to take care of our environment, and take care of ourselves.

- When we are lacking any element at all, we are lacking more than one element. There is no one who has ever lacked just one element.

- Vegetarian foods have a vibratory rate that must be balanced with an appropriate peaceful and low-key lifestyle.

- None of the diseases will come upon you if you live the laws that have been given you to live by. The spiritual laws of the universe are just as inviolable as the physical and natural laws.

Even in a logical (vs spiritual sense), a person who knows that all life comes from the Almighty knows that these statements demonstrate that He wants us, his children, to live in harmony with creation and to be healthy. How do we know? He says so in His Word; 3 John 2 says, "Beloved, I wish above all things that you would prosper and be in health, even as your soul prospers." Just like any loving parent, He equips us with everything we need to accomplish this.

In fact, He gave us a body that can heal itself of almost anything, if only we obey His instructions about how to equip the body to activate and optimize its self-healing ability. We've all witnessed the power of the human body to heal itself because everyone has cut themselves at some point or another in their lifetime. And

Any disease is simply malfunctioning cells to one degree or another, which means the root of the problem is systemic. It's your entire body reacting in a particular way.

what happened when we cut ourselves? The cut scabbed over; it healed. Perhaps we put a bandage on it to help it heal. Did the bandage heal the finger? No. The body healed itself.

The same thing happens if something is broken on the inside of the body. If a bone is broken that requires wearing a cast, does the cast heal the bone? No. The body heals itself on the inside, just as it can heal a cut that can be seen with the naked eye on the outside. So, if the body can heal itself both on the outside and the inside, and we have no trouble believing that our body can self-heal a cut, a broken bone, or even the flu or a cold, why do we doubt that we can heal ourselves of more serious ailments? Maybe it's because we have frightening names for disease; maybe that's what makes it so hard to believe that our bodies can overcome such things.

Maybe instead of calling a malignant tumor "cancer"

we should call it a "potentially reversible cellular malfunction", which is, in plain language, exactly what it is. Even mysterious sounding ailments are, really, just ailments using Latin and Greek terms to maintain a consistent nomenclature. Consider the word "fibromyalgia". The Latin term "fibro" means fibrous tissue (tendons and ligaments). "Myalgia" is derived from the Greek term "myos", meaning muscles, and "algos", which is another Greek term meaning pain. In essence, the grandiose term "fibromyalgia" means nothing more than pain in the muscles, tendons, and ligaments.

Simple or complicated, whether termed as a disease or a condition, everybody seems to have one or more Western world ailments afflicting their body — high blood pressure, cancer, diabetes, high cholesterol, stroke, adrenal fatigue, etc. There are many different names for disease, but it doesn't matter what we call it, because *all* diseases are all the same thing.

Any disease is simply malfunctioning cells to one degree or another, which means the root of the problem is systemic. It's your entire body reacting in a particular way. What I mean is, cutting out or otherwise treating the problem rarely (if ever) addresses the cause of the problem. We need to stop being fixated on localized symptoms and look at the bigger picture. We need to ask, "What is going on in the body on a systemic, holistic level that is causing certain cells to malfunction in the first place?"

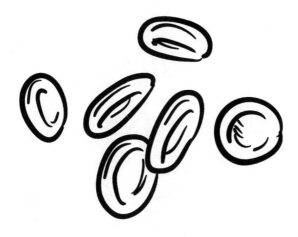

The Bible states that the Almighty's commands, though many, are summarized in just two statements: "Love God, and love people" (Matthew 22:37-40). Likewise, the cause of cellular malfunction (though the details are varied and complicated) can be summarized into two reasons: Toxicity and deficiency. In a nutshell, toxicity drags the immune system down, and nutritional deficiency starves the immune system of what it needs to fight back. When there is a combination of toxicity and deficiency, disease can take hold.

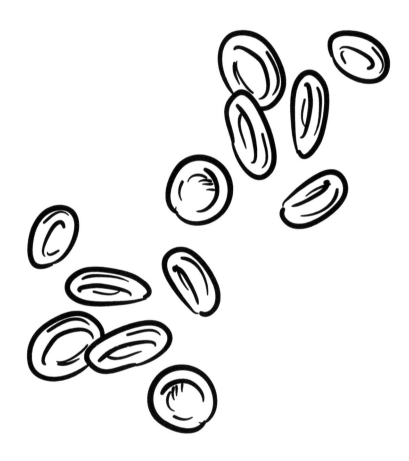

# TOXICITY: HIDDEN DANGERS

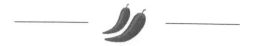

There are many sources of toxicity, including but not limited to:

- Air, water, and soil pollutants

- Chemicals in personal care products

- Dental work (fillings)

- Over-the-counter and prescription drugs

- Heavy metals (arsenic, lead, mercury, cadmium, aluminum)

- Flame retardants in clothing and furniture Bisphenol-A (BPA) from plastics

- Non-stick cookware

- Electromagnetic frequencies (EMF) from cell phones, microwaves, smart meters, and electrical towers

- Unconfessed sins, anxiety, anger, worry, resentment, bitterness, grudges

- Hurried lifestyles

- Imbalanced work/home life

- Toxic food

I'm sure you can identify with several things on this list — maybe ALL of them! One of the things on this list that surprises a lot of people is the toxin of electromagnetic frequencies (EMF). Everyone knows that cell phones pose some questionable health risks, but most people don't know that these frequencies are also emitted by many other common, everyday items in our lives. Hair dryers, for example, emit EMF. In fact, anything that is electrical and near your body has the potential to negatively impact your health. Just like a bad diet, EMF causes stress to your body, which can trigger a domino effect that can lead to disease.

> Unforgiveness will drag down your immune system, making you more prone to colds, flu, and worse. Worrying will do the same thing.

Perhaps one of the most common toxins on this list is spiritual toxins. If we don't forgive people for things they have done to us (even if they don't ask us to forgive them), those emotions create acid, just like a bad diet and EMF. Unforgiveness will drag down your immune system, making you more prone to colds, flu, and worse. Worrying will do the same thing. Just as each cigarette contributes to a smoker's risk of lung cancer, negative emotions — worrying in particular — can create a toxic snowball that can literally shorten lifespan if left unchecked.

In 2007, researchers at Purdue University concluded a study of 1,663 men, revealing that their "level and slope of neuroticism (excessive worry) interacted in their effect on mortality."[36] Essentially, the longer they continued to worry about things in their lives, the shorter their lives became. Another study in Scotland concluded after 21 years of research that "[worry] was significantly related to risk of death from cardiovascular disease." [37]

When we worry, we spark a chemical reaction in the body, creating excess free radical activity within our cells. The same thing results when we eat poorly or don't get enough exercise. The result is a general decline in health (i.e. worrying yourself sick). Sickness is, in fact, the evidence of excess free radical activity within your cells, causing toxicity that paves the way for disease.

Negative emotions (especially worry), are just not worth getting sick — or worse. In fact, worry is unbiblical. It is concern about an imminent event or uncertain outcome over which only God has control. Our Messiah himself

> When we worry, we spark a chemical reaction in the body, creating excess free radical activity within our cells. The same thing results when we eat poorly or don't get enough exercise. The result is a general decline in health (i.e. worrying yourself sick).

gave us some good advice on this point by way of a gently worded commandment: "Take therefore no thought for the morrow: for the morrow shall take thought for the things of itself." (Matthew 6:34)

When presented with an unpleasant situation, we have a choice. We can worry or trust God. Spending

> **Spending time in prayer is perhaps the most important method of reducing anxiety.**

time in prayer is perhaps the most important method of reducing anxiety. It goes back to the trust factor; by spending more time with the Almighty in prayer and meditation, your relationship with Him will grow. The more your relationship grows, the more you will learn to trust His ways, even when you can't see the light at the end of the tunnel.

At the bottom of this list is the most important and most prolific toxin: Toxic food. Now, we're not talking about pesticides on produce or even an occasional recall due to salmonella in bagged spinach. We're talking about normal, everyday, "healthy" food that is not as healthy as you think it is.

But before we get into that, we need to define what a "toxin" is. It's all about pH. We talked about the pH scale earlier in this book. It's a scale of alkalinity and acidity, measured from 0 to 14. Zero is extreme acid and 14 extreme alkaline. Seven is neutral (i.e. water), and human blood is slightly on the alkaline side, 7.38 to 7.44. Foods that create an acid ash when metabolized are going to clash with the body's alkaline nature. Now, here are some examples of acidic food, and you may be surprised.

First and foremost, meat, animal flesh any kind (red meat, white meat, fish, egg) is acid-forming. To achieve optimal health, these foods need to be drastically reduced with the ultimate goal of eliminating them completely. To replace these foods, consume more of the alkaline foods, which we'll get into a little bit later.

Dairy is also highly acid-forming. We discussed earlier in this book the irony of dairy's propensity to steal calcium from a person's bones because of the alkalinity needed to neutralize the acid created when dairy is metabolized. Again, dairy does NOT provide calcium to the body; consuming it actually creates a negative net calcium situation. This includes ALL dairy, including "healthy" yogurt. The benefits of probiotics derived from yogurt are far outweighed by the negative effects on the body due to the dairy itself. There are other ways to get probiotics including

> Refined sugar is both a
> toxin and a substance
> that causes deficiency.
> It causes deficiency by
> robbing the body of
> its nutritional stores to
> repair the damage done
> by sugar's effects

fermented foods like sauerkraut, kimchi, apple cider vinegar, and of course, naturally-derived probiotic supplements that are time-released so that they will survive the stomach environment and complete their journey to the lower portion of the colon where they do their best work. Also, a diet high in complex carbohydrates such as fruits, whole grains, and vegetables promotes the growth of Bifidobacteria (the good kind) in the large intestine. Heavy meat consumption does just the opposite.

Refined sugar, as you might imagine, is very acid-forming as well. Remember that we said that "toxicity and deficiency" were the two root causes of disease. Refined sugar is both a toxin and a substance that causes deficiency. It causes deficiency by robbing the body of its nutritional stores to repair the damage done by sugar's effects (more on this later).

Refined salt is also acid-forming. So are refined

grains and flour. You've probably heard the familiar adage most doctors advise: "Avoid any white foods". Refined salt, refined sugar, refined grains, and white rice all fall into this category. They are all acid-forming. Other refined foods include soft drinks, coffee, packaged foods containing refined ingredients (crackers, cookies, cereals), artificial sweeteners, roasted and/or salted nuts (raw nuts are OK), fried foods, refined oils, beer, wine, and spirits.

Now, you may look at this list and wonder, "What's left?" True, the "Standard American Diet" includes all of these foods and we have grown to accept them as normal. They may be considered normal, but they are certainly not health-promoting. It's no wonder that people who nourish their God-given bodies with these God-forsaken foods are prone to disease.

Acid-forming foods make the body prone to disease because they hinder the body's ability to absorb nutrients. So, they not only fill your body with empty calories, they decrease your body's ability to absorb nutrients from the healthy foods you are eating. Acid-forming foods also decrease energy production in your mitochondria, the power generators inside the body's cells. They also decrease your body's ability to repair damaged cells. So if you're trying to heal yourself from a cold or a flu or something worse, eating these is not going to help. Acid-forming foods decrease your body's ability to detoxify itself of heavy metals. These foods also increase tumor cell production. When mitochondria are completely destroyed, the cell loses its ability to convert food into energy and it dies. As one might expect, alkaline-forming foods have the opposite effect. The abundant amount of antioxidants in living food protects your cells' mitochondria from being damaged and destroyed by free radicals.

A few years ago, I had a big, strong, linebacker-sized neighbor who was 34 years old. We found out that he had esophageal cancer. His wife was a nurse, so they were committed to the standard medical route of

> Acid-forming foods also decrease energy production in your mitochondria, the power generators inside the body's cells. They also decrease your body's ability to repair damaged cells.

> The abundant amount of antioxidants in living food protects your cells' mitochondria from being damaged and destroyed by free radicals.

chemotherapy, radiation, and other allopathic modalities. I remember seeing a blog post of his during his treatments; he was so happy because he "could actually keep a hamburger down." He didn't have the knowledge that feeding his body with acid-forming foods was further destroying his already-beaten, chemically-treated body. He may have been able to keep the burger down, but it wasn't helping him. He died at 34 years old, a newly-married man. Along the way, I gently asked his wife about what was going on and asked if they had considered the type of food that he had been eating. It was not well received. However, she eventually re-married and approached me one day while we were both doing yard work. She briefly asked me about food and health. Obviously, something I had said previously had resonated with her. After our conversation that day, she never brought it up again.

Speaking of health and hospitals, I am perplexed by the nutritional protocols of a typical hospital. Why, for example, would the hospital feed sugar-laden desserts to people whose bodies are desperately absorbing nutrients to repair damage from traditional cancer therapies? I don't get it, because it's not as if doctors are ignorant of the role that sugar plays in cancer. A common cancer detection method is a PET (positron emission tomography) scan. Before undergoing the scan, the patient ingests a dye containing a type of sugar — because cancer cells require more sugar than normal cells. As the cancer cells absorb the sugar, the dye makes them stand out from normal cells, and thus they can be detected during the scan. Furthermore, sugar is now being considered to determine the level of a cancer's malignancy. In an article in the February 2016 edition of *Tomography*, researchers note that a tumor's properties can be examined by injecting a small amount of sugar into it; the more sugar the tumor consumes, the more malignant it is.[38]

Refined sugar is definitely an acidic food to avoid, but animal products are the most acid-forming of all. As we've already discussed, that includes anything that comes from an animal, whether it's meat, dairy, eggs, or even fish. If it comes from an animal, it's acidic, period — even if it's organic. It's just the nature of the beast (no pun intended, OK maybe a little intended). Bottom line: Meat and dairy are toxic because they create acidic conditions in the body, and disease thrives in an acidic

......................................

**Meat and dairy are toxic because they create acidic conditions in the body, and disease thrives in an acidic environment.**

......................................

environment. The opposite is also true: Disease cannot survive in an alkaline environment. Disease depends on acidity as its food. If disease is starved of acidity and flooded with alkalinity, it dies. These statements should come as no surprise because we know the human body can only exist in an alkaline state.

Getting back to refined sugar for a moment, I hesitate to give it a ranking of the "second-most" acid-forming food because refined sugar will bring down your immune system like nothing else. This includes white sugar, brown sugar, etc. You may already know that brown sugar is not any less refined than white sugar. Brown sugar is simply white, refined sugar that also includes molasses. Perhaps the most notorious of refined sugars, high fructose corn syrup has been linked to many health problems including heart disease, dementia, diabetes, cancer, liver failure, and of course, obesity. Keep in mind that food companies are continually attempting to downplay the negative press of this processed food ingredient.

At the time of writing this book, high fructose corn syrup was being disguised on food labels with the terms "fructose" and "fructose syrup". Fructose is a natural fruit sugar and is actually low on the glycemic index, but high fructose corn syrup (AKA "fructose" or "fructose syrup" on the labels of manufactured foods) is not the same as naturally occurring fructose. Due to processing, "fructose" as it appears in manufactured foods is only 14% fructose and has a glycemic index of 89, which is only slightly less than that of refined white sugar (92). In contrast, natural fructose has a glycemic index of 32, or almost 1/3 that of high fructose corn syrup.

Refined sugar, in general, causes more problems than many people realize. For example, it is common for people to blame dietary fat for obesity and other health problems instead of pointing the finger at sugar. The media portrays fat as the main culprit in the development of such diseases (e.g., heart disease), but sugar appears to be just as villainous.

W. D. Ringsdorf, DMD, MS, co-author of *Psychodietetics*, says that, "Sugar raises blood pressure. Sugar mixed with animal fats leads to atherosclerosis and by increasing the stickiness (viscosity) of the blood, it increases the possibility of blood clots." Refined sugar is also devoid of vitamins, minerals, or fiber, which is why I refer to it not only as a toxin but a contributor to deficiency (the perfect recipe for disease).

Refined sugar drains and leaches the body of precious vitamins and minerals through the demand that its digestion, detoxification and elimination make upon one's entire system. Taken every day, sugar produces a continuously over-acid condition, requiring more and more minerals from deep in the body to rectify the resulting acid/alkaline imbalance. Finally, in order to protect the blood, so much calcium is taken from the bones and teeth that decay and general weakening begin. This is why sugar is known to greatly increase the risk of dental decay.

Ironically, what many people don't understand is that artificial sweeteners are even worse than sugar. If you want a good sugar substitute, stevia is your best friend. Stevia is a naturally sweet plant native

> If you want a good sugar substitute, stevia is your best friend. Stevia is a naturally sweet plant native to Paraguay. Its leaves, if simply cut and sifted, can be 30 times sweeter than sugar and have no calories.

to Paraguay. Its leaves, if simply cut and sifted, can be 30 times sweeter than sugar and have no calories. The sweetness comes from calorie-free glycosides in the stevia leaf; commercially produced extracts can be 200 to 300 times sweeter than sugar. Two drops of stevia liquid or one packet of stevia powder are as sweet as two teaspoons of sugar with zero calories, zero carbs, and zero glycemic index, which means it will not raise blood sugar levels.

It is safe, non-refined, and doesn't affect the body like regular sugar does. In short, stevia has no negative effects like artificial sweeteners do. After years — in some cases, decades — of public suspicion regarding artificial sweeteners like saccharin, aspartame, and sucralose, the truth has been revealed. Thanks to whistle-blowing blogs, e-newsletters, and websites, health conscious consumers are not buying it anymore (the chemically sweetened products or the "harmless" claims). Coca-Cola and PepsiCo have taken note and are now protecting their profits by making all-natural stevia extract the next sugarless starlet. Not to mention, Japanese and Korean markets have been using stevia to sweeten soft drinks for 20 years. Furthermore, the indigenous tribes of South America have used stevia as a digestive aid and have also applied it topically for years to help wound healing. Clinical studies have shown it can increase glucose tolerance and help control blood sugar levels.[39]

Refined white salt is the next toxic food we need to discuss. Refined salt has an acidic effect on the body just like animal products and sugar. Refined salt is over 99% sodium chloride; that's not natural. Natural, unrefined sea salt or pink Himalayan salt still has all of the naturally-occurring minerals in place, which help the body deal with sodium chloride. When these minerals are removed through the refining process, refined white salt cannot give the body the tools it needs to handle sodium chloride, which is why

> Two drops of stevia liquid or one packet of stevia powder are as sweet as two teaspoons of sugar with zero calories, zero carbs, and zero glycemic index, which means it will not raise blood sugar levels.

refined salt intake leads to health problems.

In a blog article on salt and sodium, Dr. David Brownstein (a Board-Certified family physician and one of the foremost practitioners of holistic medicine) writes:

> "There is little data to support low-salt diets being effective at treating hypertension for the vast majority of people. Also, none of the studies looked at the use of unrefined sea salt, which contains many valuable vitamins and minerals such as magnesium and potassium, which are vital to maintaining normal blood pressure.

> "The conclusion that salt causes high blood pressure is based primarily on a couple of studies; neither have conclusively established a causal link between salt consumption and hypertension.

> "Low-sodium diets have been shown to cause multiple nutrient deficiencies, including depletion of minerals such as calcium, magnesium, and potassium, as well as exhausting B-vitamin stores. There are numerous studies touting the benefits

of magnesium in treating cardiovascular disorders. Adequate amounts of potassium and B-vitamins are also crucial for a healthy heart. Many studies have shown that a deficiency of minerals, particularly calcium, potassium, and magnesium is directly related to the development of heart disease as well as hypertension."

"The use of **unrefined salt will not cause elevated blood pressure**; in fact, due to its abundance of minerals, it **can actually help lower the blood pressure** in hypertensive patients." [40]

Toxic food number four is refined wheat flour. We have all heard that white bread and white flour are not good for you, but why? White flour is made by stripping all of the "good" parts of the grain kernel. Why? Because these parts tend to gum up bread manufacturing equipment. The flour is refined to make it easy to work with, then nutrients are artificially replaced, thereby making the bread "enriched" — but is this effective or even realistic? Can you simply shove nutrients back in after disrupting the delicate, natural co-factors that held those nutrients in place within the naturally-occurring grain?

You may remember the words "organic" and "inorganic" from our mineral discussion earlier in this book. For review, organic nutrients come from plants. Inorganic nutrients come from mineral salts — rocks, in other words. The nutrients that are put back into "enriched" flour are the inorganic ones. The package label may claim that the bread or flour contains "15% of your recommended daily riboflavin intake", for example. This statement is essentially true, but only if the nutrients referenced are the highly bioavailable organic nutrients. To be clear, even if the same amount of inorganic riboflavin is added back into the flour after the organic riboflavin is removed, the resulting "enriched" bread does not have the same nutritional value as the original grain.

# DEFICIENCY: TOXICITY'S PARTNER IN CRIME

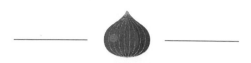

Toxicity in your body is like never changing the oil in your car. The sludge will eventually build up until the car just stops. Deficiency is like putting the wrong type of gas in your car. It won't give your car what it needs to operate properly, which exacerbates the problems caused by the dirty oil. The same thing happens in your body; wrong foods, stress, and inactivity are the toxicity. Not feeding your body with enough nutrients equals deficiency.

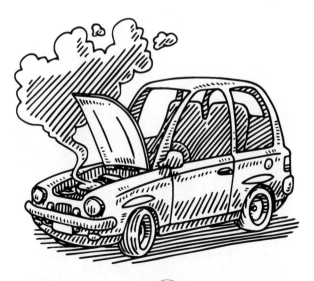

# WATER DEFICIENCY

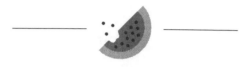

There are many different kinds of deficiencies in the body. Water, for example. Over 70% of the American population is, technically, dehydrated. Dehydration is acid-forming, causing allergies, heartburn, and needless buildup of toxins that are not being flushed out.

Even if you don't partake of water-depleting substances like alcohol, tobacco, and salty processed foods, you're likely subject to pollution, stress, and working in dry, indoor air. All of these things necessitate greater water intake than generations before us, but few of us do anything about it. As a result, dehydration creeps in, slowly and undetected, until it becomes a chronic condition. Chronic dehydration is, in fact, a major underlying cause of many common ailments in addition to causing decrements in physical, visuomotor, psychomotor,

> Water is also extremely important for energy production; for every 1% drop of water in your cells, energy production is cut by 10%.

and cognitive performance.[41]

Chronic dehydration will not give you the obvious cues of acute dehydration (dry mouth, extreme thirst, etc.). Instead, the signs of chronic dehydration manifest themselves under the guise of seemingly insignificant and/or unrelated ailments. For example, allergies (and even asthma) can be a symptom of chronic dehydration. Dehydration increases histamine levels, which causes the body to release cortisol (a stress hormone). This suppresses the production of white blood cells, making the body vulnerable to allergens. Chronic dehydration can also cause heartburn, gastroesophageal reflux disorder (GERD), joint pain (due to dried out cartilage), kidney stones, depression, among many other disorders throughout the body. Water is also extremely important for energy production; for every 1% drop of water in your cells, energy production is cut by 10%.[42] Dehydration also slows enzymatic activity, causing an imbalance in the acid/alkaline balance, which also leads to fatigue. Not to mention, when you're dehydrated, your body stops relying on fresh water coming in and begins reusing what it has (i.e. urine).

As your kidneys recycle urine, it will become more concentrated and darker in color. This, of course, increases the level of acid in your body; the darker the urine, the more acid is in your body.[43] Dehydration will also cause constipation as colon muscles contract to absorb water back into circulation. This can result in harder stool and weakened colon walls, which can develop small pockets in the colon known as diverticula (from which the condition diverticulitis is named).

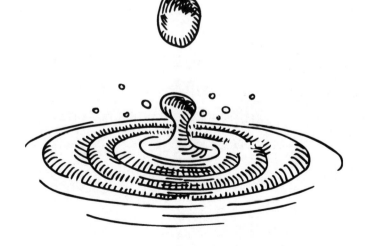

Since the blood is largely composed of water, dehydration can reduce the blood volume by reducing the water content of the blood. It can cause orthostatic hypotension (sudden low blood pressure felt as a dizzy spell when attempting to stand up), fainting, and even shock in extreme cases. Dehydration can even prevent your body from sweating enough to dilute and expel toxins.

As a result, these toxins irritate the skin and also increase the concentration of toxins inside the body; rheumatoid pain will increase, for example, in direct proportion to the concentration of toxins.
The perfect combatant to dehydration is freshly extracted, raw vegetable juice. The raw foods and juices in a whole food, plant-based diet contain abundant water in its purest form — living foods (all fruits and vegetables are sources of electrolytes too).
Of course, an abundant supply of purified water is

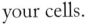

also a good idea. Here's a little tip: Drinking water a half-hour before eating will help the process of food digestion, easing its effect[44] on your cells.

# EXERCISE DEFICIENCY

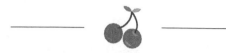

Lack of exercise, like dehydration, also increases acid formation. Lack of exercise can lead to high blood pressure, high cholesterol, and increased heart disease risk. That's why you feel so much better when you exercise! Sometimes, if you get agitated and feel tired and stressed, the best thing to do is to get some exercise.

Lack of exercise and aging also go hand in hand. If a person is inactive, muscle tone and strength can be lost, cardiovascular fitness can suffer, as can the ability to participate in sports or other physical activities. Posture will likely suffer as muscles deteriorate, back pain may settle in, and even blood pressure can begin rising. As a result, a sedentary lifestyle can lead to numerous different physical problems, like fibromyalgia. Despite the initial pain of adopting an exercise program once afflicted with fibromyalgia, exercise may be one of the most important factors for fibromyalgia sufferers to consider when searching for ways to reverse the intensity of their symptoms. Regular exercise is, in fact,

> Regular exercise is, in fact, even more important for people with fibromyalgia than for those without it as exercise raises the body's serotonin levels, which in turn stimulates endorphin production.

even more important for people with fibromyalgia than for those without it as exercise raises the body's serotonin levels, which in turn stimulates endorphin production. Endorphins are brain chemicals that act as the body's natural pain killers, whose effectiveness has been compared to morphine. Thus, with more exercise come more endorphins and the potential for less pain.

One study amplified this message by showing that fibromyalgia-like symptoms could actually be induced in sedentary individuals, but could not be replicated in individuals who were aerobically fit.[45] Another study at São Paulo Federal University in

Brazil found that inactivity not only leads to more pain, but to reduced oxygen uptake: "In patients with fibromyalgia, the anaerobic threshold and peak oxygen uptake were significantly reduced," and "…maximum heartbeat rate was significantly lower."[46] Furthermore, a finding by the American Heart Association showed that 80% of people with fibromyalgia were physically unfit in terms of maximal oxygen uptake.

Clearly, exercise is crucial for people with fibromyalgia, but there is good news. The key to reducing pain, thereby stimulating aerobic activity, may be as simple as eating your vegetables. Researchers in Finland put 18 fibromyalgia patients on a strict, low-salt, uncooked, plant-based diet for three months. Results revealed significant improvements in terms of pain, joint stiffness, and even quality of sleep. The study concluded that a "vegan diet had beneficial effects on fibromyalgia symptoms."[47]

Fibromyalgia and aging aside, even people who are quite young can seem prematurely old if they suffer from the effects of inactivity. Alternatively, exercise can actually slow aging; and it's a long lasting benefit. Not only will you feel better now, but you will be investing in a healthy and physically capable old age. Your bones will remain strong, your strength levels will stay up, your joints will stay flexible, and your outlook will be positive.

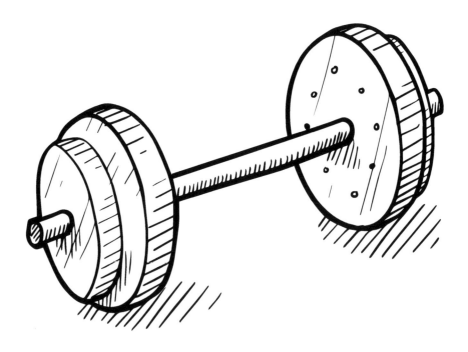

# SLEEP DEFICIENCY

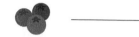

Stress due to sleep deficiency — or sleep deprivation as it is commonly known — is acid-forming just like a bad diet and inactivity. But it doesn't take much to turn things around. Just one more hour of proper sleep can decrease calcification of the arteries by 33%. How does that happen? It's really quite logical. If stress causes acid, the alkaline nature of the human body must respond the same way it does to acidic food in order to maintain its alkalinity. As you may remember from comments about dairy earlier in this book, when the body is presented with an acid-forming situation, it searches around for something alkaline to neutralize the acid. So where does it go? The bones. That's where calcium is found; the bones are the body's alkaline storehouse. It takes some calcium stores out of the bones to neutralize the acid, pushing the calcium back into the bloodstream, resulting in calcification of the arteries. By getting more sleep and reducing the acid, this domino effect can be minimized.

Sleep can also impede your weight loss goals, according to a study in the *Annals of Internal Medicine*.[48] Overweight adults were subjected to moderate caloric restriction for two 14-day intervals. They were allowed to sleep 8.5 hours per night for the first interval but only 5.5 hours for the second interval. Results showed that they lost 55% less fat when they slept fewer hours. Dr. Plaman Penev, a co-author of the study, explained it this way:

> "Sleep loss can prevent the loss of fat and make the body stingier when it comes to using fat as a fuel."

Researchers also noted that sleep loss also increases undesirable loss of lean body mass, which doesn't help the body burn energy or calories. Did you catch that? Sleep deprivation actually harms the muscle you've been working on so hard to build at the gym and does nothing for fat loss!

One of the most important aspects of getting adequate sleep is to create a sleep environment free from distractions. Similarly, your body needs to be prepared for sleep, meaning that both your brain and muscle activity need to be slowed down. Many people accomplish this by turning off the TV and shutting down the mobile phone long before they go to bed. Some take a hot bath about an hour before bedtime. It's also important to give the body enough time to properly digest food. As a general rule, most health advocates suggest at least three hours between dinner and bedtime.

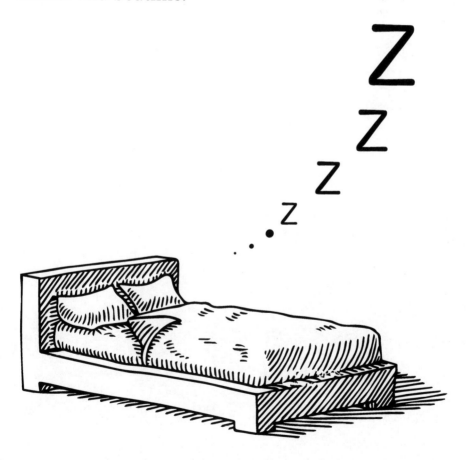

# NUTRITIONAL DEFICIENCY

## (AND HOW TO DEFEAT IT)

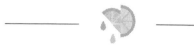

The biggest deficiency of all (and one of which you have most control) is nutritional deficiency. We eat several times every day; each time you pick up your fork is a new opportunity to replace missing nutrients. When accomplishing this goal, remember that nutrient deficiency can be caused by the same acid-forming foods that cause toxicity. Sugar, as we just discussed, is a prime example. When sugar metabolizes, it becomes a toxin. It also causes deficiency because, in order for your body to combat sugar's negative effects, your body must give up important minerals it gained from the healthy foods you've been so diligent to eat. So, that wonderful salad packed with all kinds of superfoods is wasted if you eat a sugary dessert afterwards. In order to neutralize the threat that sugar poses, the body must use all of the beneficial nutrients you just ate.

This is why I say that sugar is a double-whammy; it causes BOTH toxicity and deficiency, the two major ingredients for any and all disease.

Fortunately, there is an easy "escape route" (or "root" if you will): Stop eating acidic foods and begin eating alkaline foods. As a general rule, raw, plant-based fruits and vegetables are alkaline-forming foods. It makes perfect sense that these foods are good for us because the Almighty has adorned healthy, ripe foods with vibrant colors to which we are instinctively drawn. They taste great to the human palate, they are easy to digest, and best of all, alkaline foods are the antidote to acidity because they do not make the body fight like acidic foods do. Remember, your body is slightly alkaline, 7.38 to 7.44 on the pH scale. Your body wants to stay in that range. If you feed it alkaline foods, which are already in that range, there's no fight to maintain alkalinity. That means no free radical production, no inflammation, and thus no disease. And all the nutrients that your body is getting from those alkaline foods can be directly deposited into your bones, fed to your immune system, and pushed into all the departments that need help.

Can you get too alkaline? In theory, yes. In reality, not likely. There is so much acidity to overcome in our modern world that overdoing alkalinity to counteract it is practically impossible. It's not just about overcoming acid-forming food. As we've just discussed, lack of exercise, stress, and sleep deprivation are acid-forming, too. Even a refreshing walk outdoors has some measure of acid because of lactic acid production in your body and pollution in the air.

Avoiding toxic, acidic foods and eating alkaline foods helps the body rid itself of toxins and fat because toxins are stored in fat. If you've ever seen commercials for weight loss diet plans or a reality TV show based on extreme obesity, you'll notice that it seems like the bigger the person is, the faster the weight comes off once a proper diet and exercise plan has been implemented. And you think to yourself, "How did they do that?" Remember that toxins are stored in fat. Because there's so much fat in that person's body, once a good diet provides the body what it needs to regain health, the first thing it does is get rid of all the fat because that's where the toxins are.

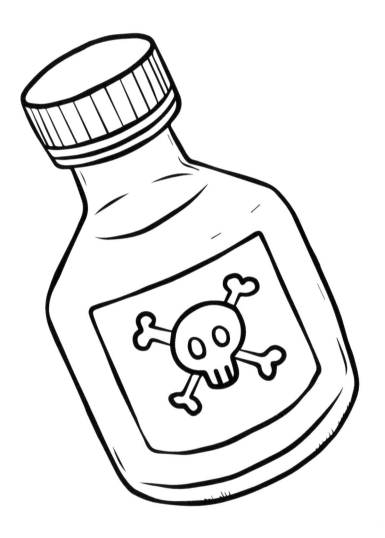

# THE ESCAPE ROOT:
# ALKALINE-FORMING FOODS

There is nothing magical or miraculous about nutritious food. What's miraculous is the self-healing body the Almighty has given you. The food is simply the fuel that empowers it; and it's more powerful than you might think.

You now have a wealth of information that can help you take yourself out of the equation of disease-related statistics — you have discovered the escape "root", the secret passage to lifelong wellness. Most people will never know what you have just learned; in fact, most people won't believe you when you try to tell them about it. Expect it, and accept it. Just like the narrow road that leads to eternal life (Matthew 7:14), you are on the narrow road that leads to physical life. And likewise, "only a few find it".

The key to this "secret passage" is, of course, the right food choices — raw, enzyme-rich, plant-based food, food that grows from the ground, the "root" (if you will) in "escape root". Now, the first thing you need to understand is that there is nothing magical or miraculous about nutritious food. What's miraculous is the self-healing body the Almighty has given you. The food is simply the fuel that empowers it; and it's more powerful than you might think.

When I worked at *The Hallelujah Diet* from 2008 to 2013, we would host plant-based dietary information seminars on the first Saturday of every month. My job was to be the MC and to help people with questions after the event. People would show up in droves despite that advertising was minimal. Some 200 to 400 people would arrive out of the woodwork, every month. It was like a scene from the movie, *The Field of Dreams*. "If you build it, they will come" the movie surmised in its most notable quote. At *The Hallelujah Diet*, it happened just like that: We put the truth out there and people came. Some were desperate for answers after doctors had given them a death sentence. Some were sick and tired of being sick and tired. Some were just curious. And then there were those who came to give their testimony.

Without fail, when Rev. George Malkmus (founder of *The Hallelujah Diet* and the main speaker at these events) would ask if there was anyone who had a healing testimony after adopting a plant-based diet, there were 10, 20, or even more who shared; different people at every event, every month. It was amazing. They would stand up to tell their testimony as I would rush to them with a cordless microphone so that everyone could hear what they had to say.

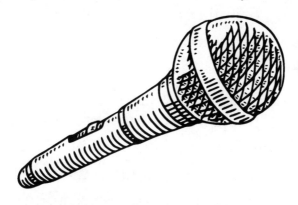

From fibromyalgia, diabetes, Lyme disease, high blood pressure, heart disease, multiple sclerosis, and even stage-4 cancer of the breast, prostate, colon, and even the brain, it didn't matter: Their symptoms were gone. Their doctors were amazed. Some even brought the before-and-after lab tests to prove the reversal of their symptoms (because lab tests don't lie). All these people did was shun the diet of the world and adopt a raw, enzyme-rich, plant-based diet.

> The most powerful weapon in a no-junk, primarily raw, plant-based diet is freshly extracted vegetable juice. This does not mean that juice in your local grocery store is the same thing, however.

As we've already discussed, the most powerful weapon in a no-junk, primarily raw, plant-based diet is freshly extracted vegetable juice. This does not mean that juice in your local grocery store is the same thing, however. (This point was mentioned earlier in this book, but it bears repeating.) By law, juice on a grocery store shelf must be preserved in some form or fashion to maintain its shelf life. Until recently, that usually meant pasteurization, which is flash heating the juice to kill the enzymes that would naturally spoil the juice after a day or so. Destroying the enzymes also destroys the juice's life force that helps the human body heal. A few years ago, some manufacturers claimed that "flash pasteurization" was better because it subjected the juice to heat for only a short period — but it still killed enzymes. Most recently, a new kind of preservation method has taken hold, which addresses the concerns of consumers smart enough to look for "cold pressed" juice. High pressure processing (HPP) is a process during which freshly sealed bottles of raw vegetable juice are put into giant water chamber where the bottles are subjected to 85,000 PSI of water pressure.

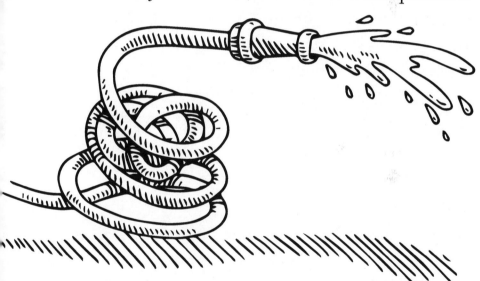

The process does create some heat, though not as much as traditional pasteurization. The pressure also damages enzymes. However, the biggest misguided assumption is that the nutrients in raw juice subjected to this kind of preservation can remain intact for the duration of the juice's shelf life. They can't. Though HPP may satisfy the FDA's requirement for preservation and satisfy the trendy consumer's desire for "cold processing", the fact remains that nutrients in raw vegetable juice begin to break down within a few days; raw juice is still best.

Again, for review, most raw vegetables and raw fruits are alkaline-forming. Most raw nuts and most raw seeds are alkaline-forming, too. Raw food is where the enzymes are, and where the enzymes are, self-healing is not far behind.

# Alkaline Foods Chart[49]

## Vegetables

Freshly extracted vegetable juices
Artichokes
Eggplant
Beets
Summer squash
Baked potato
Zucchini
Bell peppers
Okra
Broccoli
Cabbage
Stringbeans without formed beans
Asparagus
Onions
Celery
Kohlrabi
Collard greens
Parsnips
Endive
Mustard greens
Kale
Winter squash
Sweet potatoes/Yams
Snow peas
Carrots, organic
Cucumbers
Brussels sprouts
Cauliflower
Mushrooms

## Fruits

Blackberries
Nectarines
Strawberries
Persimmon
Raspberries
Tangerines
Limes
Papaya
Pineapple
Watermelon
Cantaloupe/Honeydew
Raisins
Grapes
Blueberries
Oranges
Apples
Cherries
Apricots
Grapefruit
Avocado
Olives, green
Banana
Pears/Peaches
Lemons

## Nuts, Seeds, Legumes, Herbs and Spices

Black pepper
Lentils
Cashews
Basil
Garlic
Cilantro
Cinnamon
Soy sauce
Chestnuts
Sea salt
Ginger root
Pumpkin seeds
Parsley
Almonds
Bay leaf
Cayenne pepper
Sesame/Sunflower seeds

## Drinks

Ionized alkaline water
Ginger tea
Grapefruit juice
Pineapple juice
Apple juice
Grape juice
Orange juice
Green/Herbal tea

You'll notice vegetable juices at the top of this list of alkaline foods — this is because they are the most important alkaline food. Juicing concentrates alkaline forming nutrients into an easily digestible form (as discussed earlier in this book). Juicing feeds your body quickly and efficiently with as little digestive effort as possible because juicing separates the juice from the fiber and almost all the nutrition is in the juice. That's how eight ounces of juice can contain all the nutrition of a whole pound of carrots.

Foods that grow from the ground are not the only sources of alkalinity, however. Plants that grow in the sea can be even more powerful. Sea vegetables are an amazing class of alkaline-forming organisms (algae). They offer the broadest range of minerals of any food because they are surrounded by seawater, which contains virtually all of the same minerals found in human blood — it is literally the lifeblood of Earth itself! As such, it's not difficult to comprehend that sea vegetables are a crucial source of human nutrition. They are an excellent source of iodine, a very good source of vitamin K, riboflavin (B2), folate (folic acid), calcium, iron, magnesium, manganese, and are a good source of dietary fiber, vitamin C, pantothenic acid (B5), zinc, and copper.

Sea vegetables and their blue-green algae cousins are not new to the human diet. Civilizations around the world have used them for centuries and even millennia; Asian cultures have been using them for thousands of years. Sea vegetables have always been a part of everyday Japanese diets, while the Chinese reserved them for honored guests and royalty.

African peoples living near Lake Chad have been consuming spirulina blue-green algae since the beginning of habitation in the area. Sifted from the lake then dried on rocks, spirulina supplies these people with the highest protein content of any edible living thing on earth (including animal flesh). Hemp's celebrated 50% protein content pales in comparison to spirulina's 65%-71%. Furthermore, a study in 2005 found that spirulina protects against hay fever and a 2007 study found that volunteers taking 4.5 grams of spirulina a day exhibited significant improvement in cholesterol and blood pressure.[50]

Another advantage of sea vegetables is their rich source of iodine; the human body cannot live without it. Sea vegetables are creation's richest sources of iodine, and kelp is the most abundant, iodine-rich sea vegetable. These brown algae can have up to 8000 parts per million (ppm) iodine. Iodine helps organs to function more effectively and is especially important for the regulation of the thyroid gland. The thyroid needs iodine to function in its capacity to affect nerve health, bone formation, reproduction, speech, mental state, and more. Brown kelp has been used to treat goiter, an enlargement of the thyroid gland caused by a lack of iodine, since medieval times. Nori tends to have the least iodine of the commonly eaten sea vegetables at 15 ppm.

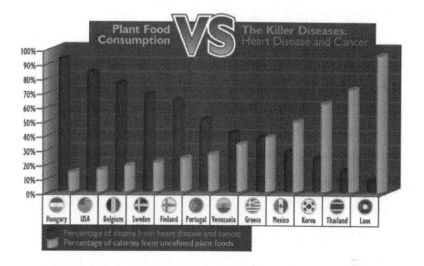

**Chart courtesy of The Hallelujah Diet.** Sources: *World Health Statistics Annual 1994-1998*; Food and Agriculture Organization of the United Nations, Statistical database food balance sheets, 1961-1999; National Institutes of Health. Global cancer rates, cancer death rates among 50 countries, 1986-1999.

Here is something very interesting. Take a look at this chart and notice the inverse correlation between consumption of plant-based foods and the rates of heart disease and cancer. The light grey bars represent the consumption level of alkaline-forming, plant-based foods. The dark grey bars represent the rates of heart disease and cancer. At the far left side, we see that the people in Hungary and the USA have a great percentage of deaths as a result of heart disease and a very small percentage of dietary calories in the form of unrefined, plant-based foods. Now consider the opposite side of this chart. The country of Laos has a very high percentage of calories coming from plant-based foods and they have almost no heart disease and cancer. The numbers don't lie. Now, for argument's sake, let's consider a very popular, so-called healthy diet like the Mediterranean diet. There is, in fact, a Mediterranean country on this chart — Greece is right in the middle. According to this chart, people in Greece generally get about 40% of their calories from plant-based food, but their percentage of death from heart disease and cancer is also about 40%. I don't know about you, but I'd rather be on the Laotian diet than the Mediterranean diet.

The bottom line is that the miracle of self-healing is within you. The Almighty put it there; it's been part of the human body since the beginning of time, but you have to activate it. It's up to you to make it happen. You make the choices. In Deuteronomy 30:19, the Almighty gave the Israelites a choice between life and death and encouraged them to choose life, in a spiritual sense. Today, I want to challenge you with that same choice in a physical sense. Your health is the result of choices you make every day. Choose life — the escape "root" of a plant-based diet, the secret passage to lifelong wellness.

# REFERENCES

[1]Wadhwa R, Singh R, Gao R, Shah N, Widodo N, Nakamoto T, Ishida Y, Terao K,
Kaul SC. Water extract of Ashwagandha leaves has anticancer activity: identification of an active component and its mechanism of action. PLoS One. 2013
Oct 10;8(10):e77189.

[2]Zarai Z, Ben Chobba I, Ben Mansour R, Békir A, Gharsallah N, Kadri A. Essential oil of the leaves of Ricinus communis L.: in vitro cytotoxicity and antimicrobial properties. Lipids Health Dis. 2012 Aug 13;11:102.

[3]Pandey A, Kaushik A, Wanjari M, Dey YN, Jaiswal BS, Dhodi A. Antioxidant and anti-inflammatory activities of Aerva pseudotomentosa leaves. Pharm Biol. 2017
Dec;55(1):1688-1697.

[4]Mathers JC, Coxhead JM, Tyson J. Nutrition and DNA repair--potential molecular mechanisms of action. Curr Cancer Drug Targets. 2007 Aug;7(5):425-31. Review.

[5]Azqueta A, Slyskova J, Langie SA, O'Neill Gaivão I, Collins A. Comet assay to measure DNA repair: approach and applications. Front Genet. 2014 Aug 25;5:288.

[6]Ames BN, Elson-Schwab I, Silver EA. High-dose vitamin therapy stimulates variant enzymes with decreased coenzyme binding affinity (increased K(m)):
relevance to genetic disease and polymorphisms. Am J Clin Nutr. 2002 Apr;75(4):616-58. Review.

[7]Suicide by Sugar by Nancy Appleton, PhD and G.N. Jacobs.

[8]Seckbach, Joseph (editor) (2004). Origins: Genesis, Evolution

and Diversity of Life. Dordrecht, The Netherlands: Kluwer Academic Publishers. p. 20.

[9]www.nutritionfacts.org

[10]www.calorieking.com

[11]Thiel, Robert J. Naturopathy for the 21st Century. Warsaw, IN: Whitman, 2000. Print.

[12]Bae S, Ulrich CM, Neuhouser ML, Malysheva O, Bailey LB, Xiao L, Brown EC, Cushing-Haugen KL, Zheng Y, Cheng TY, Miller JW, Green R, Lane DS, Beresford SA, Caudill MA. Plasma choline metabolites and colorectal cancer risk in the Women's Health Initiative Observational Study. Cancer Res. 2014 Dec 15;74(24):7442-52.

[13]Keum N, Lee DH, Marchand N, Oh H, Liu H, Aune D, Greenwood DC, Giovannucci EL. Egg intake and cancers of the breast, ovary and prostate: a dose-response meta-analysis of prospective observational studies. Br J Nutr. 2015 Oct 14;114(7):1099-107.

[14]Cornelli U. Treatment of Alzheimer's disease with a cholinesterase inhibitor combined with antioxidants. Neurodegener Dis. 2010;7(1-3):193-202.

[15]Khaw KT, Bingham S, Welch A, Luben R, Wareham N, Oakes S, Day N. Relation between plasma ascorbic acid and mortality in men and women in EPIC-Norfolk prospective study: a prospective population study. European Prospective Investigation into Cancer and Nutrition. Lancet. 2001 Mar 3;357(9257):657-63.

[16]Kromhout D, Bloemberg B, Feskens E, Menotti A, Nissinen A. Saturated fat, vitamin C and smoking predict long-term population all-cause mortality rates in

the Seven Countries Study. Int J Epidemiol. 2000 Apr;29(2):260-5.

[17]Padayatty SJ, Riordan HD, Hewitt SM, Katz A, Hoffer LJ, Levine M. Intravenously administered vitamin C as cancer therapy: three cases. CMAJ. 2006 Mar 28;174(7):937-42.

[18]Riordan HD, Riordan NH, Jackson JA, Casciari JJ, Hunninghake R, González MJ, Mora EM, Miranda-Massari JR, Rosario N, Rivera A. Intravenous vitamin C as a chemotherapy agent: a report on clinical cases. P R Health Sci J. 2004 Jun;23(2):115-8.

[19]Agarwal R, Agarwal C, Ichikawa H, Singh RP, Aggarwal BB. Anticancer potential of silymarin: from bench to bed side. Anticancer Res. 2006 Nov-Dec;26(6B):4457-98.

[20]Lazzeroni M, Guerrieri-Gonzaga A, Gandini S, Johansson H, Serrano D, Cazzaniga M, Aristarco V, Puccio A, Mora S, Caldarella P, Pagani G, Pruneri G, Riva A, Petrangolini G, Morazzoni P, DeCensi A, Bonanni B. A Presurgical Study of Oral Silybin-Phosphatidylcholine in Patients with Early Breast Cancer. Cancer Prev Res (Phila). 2016 Jan;9(1):89-95.

[21]Nambiar DK, Rajamani P, Deep G, Jain AK, Agarwal R, Singh RP. Silibinin Preferentially Radiosensitizes Prostate Cancer by Inhibiting DNA Repair Signaling. Mol Cancer Ther. 2015 Dec;14(12):2722-34.

[22]Bhatia V, Falzon M. Restoration of the anti-proliferative and anti-migratory effects of 1,25-dihydroxyvitamin D by silibinin in vitamin D-resistant colon cancer cells. Cancer Lett. 2015 Jul 1;362(2):199-207.

[23]Mahabir S, Schendel K, Dong YQ, Barrera SL, Spitz MR, Forman MR. Dietary alpha-, beta-, gamma- and delta-tocopherols in lung cancer risk. Int J Cancer.

2008 Sep 1;123(5):1173-80.

[24]Sze Ue Luk1, Wei Ney Yap, Yung-Tuen Chiu et al. Gamma-tocotrienol as an effective agent in targeting prostate cancer stem cell-like population. International Journal of Cancer, 2011. Vol 128, No 9, p 2182-2191.

[25]Nesaretnam K, Teoh HK, Selvaduray KR, Bruno RS, Ho E. Modulation of cell growth and apoptosis response in human prostate cancer cells supplemented with tocotrienols. Eur. J. Lipid Sci. Technol. 2008, 110, 23-31.

[26]Conte C, Floridi A, Aisa C, Piroddi M, Floridi A, Galli F. Gamma-tocotrienol metabolism and antiproliferative effect in prostate cancer cells. Ann N Y Acad Sci. 2004 Dec;1031:391-4.

[27]Thiel, Robert J. Naturopathy for the 21st Century. Warsaw, IN: Whitman, 2000. Print.

[28]Talalay P, Fahey JW, Healy ZR, et al. Sulforaphane mobilizes cellular defenses that protect skin against damage by UV radiation. Proceedings of the National Academy of Sciences of the United States of America. 2007;104(44):17500-17505.

[29]The China Study by T. Colin Campbell (pp 30-31, 308)

[30]Prior IA, Davidson F, Salmond CE, Czochanska Z. Cholesterol, coconuts, and diet on Polynesian atolls: a natural experiment: the Pukapuka and Tokelau island studies. Am J Clin Nutr. 1981 Aug;34(8):1552-61.

[31]Welch AA, Shakya-Shrestha S, Lentjes MAH, Wareham NJ, Khaw KT. Dietary intake and status of n-3 polyunsaturated fatty acids in a population of fish-eating and non-fish-eating meat-eaters, vegetarians, and vegans and the precursor-product ratio of a-linolenic acid to long-chain n-3 polyunsaturated fatty acids: results from the EPIC-Norfolk cohort. Am J Clin Nutr.

2010;92:1040-1051.

[32]Lands WE, Morris A, Libelt B. Quantitative effects of dietary polyunsaturated fats on the composition of fatty acids in rat tissues. Lipids. 1990;25:505-516.

[34]Simopoulous AP. The importance of the omega-6/omega-3 fatty acid ratio in cardiovascular disease and other chronic diseases. Exp Biol Med (Maywood). 2008;233:674-688.

[35]Jensen, Bernard. The Chemistry of Man. Winona Lake, IN: Whitman, 2007. Print.

[36]Mroczek DK, Spiro A 3rd. Personality change influences mortality in older men. Psychol Sci. 2007 May;18(5):371-6.

[37]Shipley BA, Weiss A, Der G, Taylor MD, Deary IJ. Neuroticism, extraversion, and mortality in the UK Health and Lifestyle Survey: a 21-year prospective cohort study. Psychosom Med. 2007 Dec;69(9):923-31.

[38]Peter C.M. van Zijl et al. Dynamic Glucose-Enhanced (DGE) MRI: Translation to Human Scanning and First Results in Glioma Patients. Tomography, February 2016

[39]KU Leuven. "Researchers unravel how stevia controls blood sugar levels." ScienceDaily. ScienceDaily, 11 April 2017.

[40]www.celticseasaltblog.com/articles/salt-articles/salt-your-way-to-health/

[41]Grandjean AC, Grandjean NR. Dehydration and Cognitive Performance. J Am Coll Nutr. 2007 Oct;26(5 Suppl):549S 554S.

[42]Dehydration's Hidden Symptoms, Brian D. Foltz and Joe

Ferrara, PhD

[43]Dangers of Chronic Dehydration by Albert Grazia, MS, ND

[44]Your Body's Many Cries for Water by F. Batmanghelidj, MD

[45]www.spine-health.com

[46]J Rheumatol. 2002 Feb;29(2):353-7.

[47]Scand J Rheumatol. 2000;29(5):308-13.

[48]Nedeltcheva AV, Kilkus JM, Imperial J, Schoeller DA, Penev PD. Insufficient Sleep Undermines Dietary Efforts to Reduce Adiposity. Ann Intern Med. 2010;153:435-441.

[49]www.betterbones.com/alkaline-balance/alkaline-forming-foods/

[50]Torres-Duran, Ferreira-Hermosillo, & Juarez-Oropeza. (2007). Antihyperlipemic and antihypertensive effects of Spirulina maxima in an open sample of Mexican population: A preliminary report. Lipids in Health and Disease. 6, 33

# NOTES

# NOTES

Made in the USA
Middletown, DE
17 April 2018